D1457648

A Doctor's Tales

Lawrence R. Brownlee, M.D.

PAGE PUBLISHING, INC.
New York, NY

First originally published by Page Publishing, Inc.
2018

ISBN 978-1-64350-520-6 (Paperback)
ISBN 978-1-64424-306-0 (Hardcover)
ISBN 978-1-64350-522-0 (Digital)

Printed in the United States of America

This book is lovingly dedicated to my wife and daughters who, for many years, gracefully tolerated my late homecomings and frequent absences while I cared for patients and attended hospital meetings and continuing medical education seminars.

$\mathcal{C}$ontents

Preface

T HERE HAVE BEEN countless scholarly case histories authored by doctors for doctors. However, few have been written by private practice physicians and worded in language accessible to the general public.

People in all walks of life have demonstrated an insatiable appetite for information about anything medical or surgical. And in recent years, the lay press has attempted to assuage that hunger with an increasing number of fact-based case histories published across print, electronic, and social media. Many of these pieces are written by journalists, based on review of current medical journals or interviews with researchers. While their writing skills are superior to mine, I believe a doctor in general practice with forty years of daily patient encounters is in a unique position to relate many entertaining and informative tales.

This collection of case histories was inspired by real events. Each tale is told from my own recollections, those of my receptionist, and my nurse, and from actual chart notes made at the time.

The whole range of human emotions—fear, pain, anger, sorrow, joy, and love—are featured in these stories. But while I wrote these stories with an eye to their entertainment value, I also felt an obligation to educate the reader about the conditions described and to persuade others of the value of early consultation, diagnosis, and treatment. I hope to encourage my readers to have a heightened awareness of symptoms that should motivate them to visit their doctors promptly. In that way, perhaps this book will change behavior and save a few lives.

For the sake of patient privacy, I have used pseudonyms and made minor alterations in person, time, and place. These changes have not affected the facts as observed and recorded.

*A*cknowledgments

To Eileen, my loyal receptionist—and much of the time my nurse, phlebotomist, and billing clerk—I owe the most praise for her encouragement, suggestions for interesting patient's stories, and help with rewrites.

Similarly, Vicky, my back office assistant, deserves thanks for her help and support.

Donna, a patient and published novelist, I credit with the motivation to get me started.

Mary Agnes, a patient, corrected all my first rough dictations, a multiyear task.

I must also thank Terri, my typist. And many thanks to Anne, my copy editor, who endeavored to make a writer of me.

CHAPTER 1

The Lady With One Breast

> *We are apt to shut our eyes against a painful truth. . . . For my part, whatever anguish of spirit it may cost, I am willing to know the whole truth—to know the worst and to provide for it.*
>
> —Patrick Henry

E VERY MORNING IN the shower, as she rubbed the bar of soap over the raw, fleshy mass that used to be her right breast and felt the enlarging lumps under her arm, Mrs. Smith anguished over her failure to seek help long ago for this disease that was now consuming her.

As was her practice, she covered the area with a large Telfa gauze pad, and donned one of several long-sleeved blouses she had purchased to conceal the swelling of her arm. Then she put the thought of it and the pain out of her mind for another day.

Mrs. Smith was a fifty-nine-year-old lady who was enjoying a long, happy marriage. In recent years, she and her husband had merely been good companions, no longer engaging in sexual relations due to her husband's erectile dysfunction. They even slept separately which made him less aware of his wife's condition.

Their Single Mom daughter had died suddenly, and the Smiths were still grieving her loss. The court had given these grandparents the responsibilities and challenges of raising their daughter's two young children. Mrs. Smith was enjoying that duty. On the rare occasion when she allowed her thoughts to drift to the increasing severity of her breast disease, she worried about the future of these motherless children.

One morning at breakfast, Mr. Smith noticed that his wife's right hand appeared swollen. When he mentioned it, she said, "Oh, it's nothing. I fell and hurt my arm, but it's getting better."

Concerned, he rolled up her sleeve, only to discover that her entire right upper limb was nearly double its usual size. She was reluctant to let him look beyond her shoulder. Suddenly, he recalled that for many weeks now his wife had worn long-sleeved blouses exclusively, something she had never done before. He now realized that she had been concealing some profound health problem from him.

Being a man of action, he made an immediate appointment, over her protestations, for a visit with me, his regular physician, and brought her in, stating she had been hiding a serious health issue that was now causing pain in her chest and right arm.

According to my nurse, who brought the patient into an examining room, Mrs. Smith seemed reluctant to remove her blouse to don our paper examining gown in the nurse's presence.

After entering the room and introducing myself, I sat down and praised the love and concern shown to her by her husband, in bringing her to a doctor at once. Before asking her to tell me the whole story of her arm and breast problem, I reviewed her entire past medical history. That put her at ease a little.

It soon became apparent that she had found a lump in her right breast a very long time ago, but instead of seeking help had shut out the painful truth from her mind. In recent months, the disease had progressed. The growth enlarged, the skin discolored, and then broke open. It soon became macerated, or soft, and began to slough off in her daily showers. When she rubbed soap over the hollow that was gradually forming in her right breast, she could feel that this disease was eating away at her breast tissue. That had led to exposure, bacterial infection, and an ongoing secretion of pus. More recently, she had developed several large tender lumps in the axilla, or armpit, on the same side.

Upon examining the patient, I found that her entire right arm and hand had massive edema, or swelling. There was an irregular mass occupying the base of the right breast, visible through a three-inch-diameter hollow devoid of skin in the upper outer part of the breast. The raw flesh had become deeply infected and was exuding thick, discolored, putrid, malodorous mucus. The skin surrounding the entire breast region, and the right chest wall was markedly pinkish-red, indicative of inflammatory carcinoma, complicated by a spreading cellulitis, or infection of the surrounding skin.

Palpation with a gloved hand, pressing gently and deeply with my fingers to feel the underlying structures, revealed the tumor mass to be firm and immobile. The area where the skin had broken down showed the muscles of the chest wall underlying the breast to be involved with the disease, too. A grape-like cluster of enlarged lymph nodes associated with this cancer was present in the right axilla. This woman's diseased breast was the most far-advanced cancer I ever encountered in my entire medical career.

Further palpation of her opposite breast revealed a small mass that could be a cyst, a benign tumor, or—more likely—an early cancer tumor as well since the greatest risk factor for breast cancer is a history of having had a prior breast cancer.

I explained to Mrs. Smith that cancer cells from carcinoma of the breast had invaded the lymphatic system of channels and nodes under her arm, blocking the flow of lymphatic fluid returning from her hand to the upper body, and causing edema of her arm and shoulder.

Mrs. Smith proceeded to recount tearfully how she had initially used denial, like Scarlett O'Hara: "I won't worry about that today, I'll worry about that tomorrow." But lately, she had awakened to the fact that she had cancer lying within her breast, trying to destroy it, and her. Even so, she continued to hide her head in the sand by avoiding looking at that part of her body or even thinking about the consequences of her inaction.

On a few occasions when she was alone at home, she would cry at her plight. But most of the time, she would dismiss it from her mind, carrying on with her normal activities of daily living and raising her two grandchildren.

I felt indescribable sadness and empathy for this incredibly neglectful but courageous lady.

My initial treatment was to lavage, or wash, and rinse the open cavity in the right pectoral area with sterile saline solution, then apply a film of antibiotic ointment and a nonstick Telfa dressing.

In my counseling of her afterward, Mrs. Smith took great comfort upon hearing that a great deal could be done to help her, especially with the wound closure; her daily cleansing and bandaging had become a dreadful ordeal.

She refused the suggestion of hospitalization, so initially, I administered a potent, broad-spectrum antibiotic intramuscularly [IM], followed by a prescription for high-dose oral antibiotics for ten days.

This treatment eliminated the infection and foul secretions, paving the way for surgical excision of the tumor mass, followed by skin grafting by a plastic surgeon to cover the gaping wound. Following this, chemotherapy and radiation therapy would be considered for palliation, and to shrink the tumor bulk.

While I tried to hold out as much hope as possible for the patient, I suspected that the disease process had gone so far that it probably had infiltrated locally into the intercostal muscles between the ribs and on into the lung. It also may have metastasized, traveling through the bloodstream to distant organs. If so, the overall expected outcome was bleak.

To survey the full extent of the disease, computerized axial tomography (CAT or CT) scans of the thorax and abdomen were required. They showed cancer invasion of the pleural cavity between the lung and the ribs, but it had not yet invaded the pleural capsule enclosing the lung itself, or any other organs. A nuclear bone scan revealed no spread of the breast malignancy to any bones. These revelations made the prognosis (outlook for the future) a little brighter, although a mammogram of the opposite breast confirmed the presence of a small but early malignant tumor there, too.

I referred Mrs. Smith to a team of my favorite skilled specialists: a radiologist, a surgeon, a pathologist, an oncologist, and a plastic surgeon.

All agreed that because of her denial and the long delay in searching out treatment, the likelihood of the patient surviving for more than six months was slim to none. In such cases, chemotherapy, with its undesirable side effects, was not usually offered.

It fell upon the oncologist, with his training and experience, to decide how much "good time" could be bought for a patient with her prognosis, and whether chemotherapy would be worthwhile.

In that era, chemo was only palliative, or life prolonging, not curative. The oncologist decided that because this woman and her elderly husband had the sole responsibility as surrogate parents for their grandchildren, and because of Mrs. Smith's now-positive attitude and her determination to see her grandchildren into young adulthood, he would recommend aggressive treatment.

In a matter of days, Mrs. Smith underwent surgical biopsy of the breast tumor. This sampling of the tumor growth would make it possible for the pathologist, a specialist in the structure of organs and tissues, to classify the type and stage of her cancer. That information assisted the team in formulating the following treatment program.

After discussions with the patient and her husband, Mrs. Smith underwent a course of intravenous (IV) chemotherapy, followed later by a course of external beam radiation. To everyone's delight, those treatments consolidated and diminished the bulk of the malignant tumor significantly.

Following the chemo and radiation, the breast surgeons performed a radical mastectomy on the right, completely excising all cancer tissue, infected tissue, remaining healthy breast tissue, and associated lymph nodes in the armpit. A simple lumpectomy to cut out the cancerous tumor with a rim of apparently healthy tissue surrounding it was done for the small tumor of the left breast. As the final step, the plastic surgeon scrubbed in to join the general surgeons to cover the large area devoid of breast and skin, utilizing modern grafting techniques to shave a thin layer of donor skin from the patient's thigh. Mrs. Smith could have opted for further plastic procedures at a later date to restore a normal-looking breast with silicone augmentation, but because of her age decided not to.

Post-op, the surgical sites, the skin graft, and the donor sites healed well. The healthy new skin that covered the defect where the diseased breast had been made personal hygiene an easy matter for Mrs. Smith. She soon returned to her normal activities of daily living.

Approximately one year later there was a recurrence of multiple small tumors on the skin of the chest wall. Following consultation with the experts on the team, a second course of radiation therapy was administered, which she tolerated well, and the tumors regressed.

At this point in the strategy, Mrs. Smith was feeling and looking quite well. During the years that followed, she was monitored closely, and responded well to additional treatments as they became available.

She confounded her specialists by miraculously remaining alive, well, and productive for at least three more years that I was aware of. Then the Smiths moved out of the area, and I lost track of them.

The Smiths firmly believed it was God's plan for this lady and her husband to continue raising their grandchildren into young adulthood before their grandmother passed away.

This patient represents only one of many similar women with cancer phobia I encountered in my medical practice over the years. Her case had a happier ending than most, but serves to illustrate the danger of irrational fear of cancer.

If you the reader or your doctor should find a breast lump, or a mammogram should reveal one, don't despair, don't be fearful! Instead, follow Patrick Henry's admonition.

Medical science is getting close to being able to prevent breast cancer but is not yet there. Early diagnosis, however, is.

The most important defensive measures are the following:

- Monthly self-examination, since 80 percent of breast tumors are found by patients, not doctors.
- Annual female organ physical exam and mammography.

Most doctors send postcards to remind patients when their annual checkups are due. During these checkups, the physician typically will teach the best way to self-check one's breasts, while reminding patients of the importance of doing it monthly. The doctor will also prescribe a screening mammogram, if due. But some patients never take the prescription to the imaging facility. Breast cancer is curable only if found early enough!

Some women may hesitate to have annual mammograms done because they have heard about radiation danger from mammography, but it is in fact negligible. In my opinion, the lay press overstates the risk, especially when compared to the heartbreaking grief of the prolonged illness and premature death that failing to obtain mammography can bring.

Many insurance organizations provide no-charge mammography as part of their preventive health programs. Even if a woman has no insurance, the cost of a screening mammogram typically varies between $80 to $100, a small price to pay for peace of mind, breast preservation, and a long life.

State-of-the-art mammography detects 85 percent of all hidden breast cancers that are not palpable.

If a woman discovers a lump in her breast, or her doctor finds one, or a mammogram reveals a suspicious cluster of specks of calcium, it is understandable for her to be frightened, or even overwhelmed. Often due to these emotions of anxiety and fear the diagnosis has evoked, the patient will not truly hear her doctor's attempt to give her reassurance that the lump or other findings may not necessarily be malignant. In fact, the majority of breast lumps prove to be noncancerous and benign.

Women care deeply about the loss of a breast, and after they become aware of a problem that could result in a mastectomy, they find it difficult not to conjure up a mental image of their postsurgical appearance. It is essential for women to know that with early diagnosis, breast-preservation surgery (lumpectomy versus the old radical mastectomy), usually followed by chemotherapy and/or radiation therapy, is now the accepted treatment for stages I and II of breast cancer, when the cancerous cells are still confined to a relatively small area within the breast. Even if a malignancy is more advanced when it is detected, treatment options are available that can provide for hope and acceptable outcomes.

If you should become aware of or be given the unhappy news of a possible problem with your breast, please do not live in denial, as did Mrs. Smith. Let Patrick Henry be your role model: instead of shutting your eyes to the painful truth, learn the whole truth about your disease and then provide for it by taking control of your destiny.

Educate yourself about your particular type of malignancy by asking questions of your doctor, surgeon, and treatment team. Read all you can find on the subject, preferably authored by medical professionals. Learn and become an "expert." There is always time to do this before you must make decisions about the options presented to you.

Your physician can put you in touch with a breast cancer support group, led by women who have themselves experienced breast cancer. They will soon help you realize that you will survive. They will help you deal with your anger and fear, rather than suppressing it, will help you overcome the depression that often sets in, and will help you retain your sense of humor.

Enlist the aid of your husband, your best friend, or a close relative to accompany you to keep your spirits up on every visit to your doctors and for treatments.

Most importantly, develop a positive mental attitude and keep your faith. Spiritual strength will help see you through your ordeal.

How often do you need a mammogram? Unbelievably, there is no consensus among cancer organizations. Unfortunately, the current Obamacare recommendations (promulgated by academics and politicians with budgets in mind) say you are to wait until age fifty for the first mammogram, then every two years until age seventy. Generally speaking, socialized medicine advocates, like former President Obama, most Democrats, and AARP, who push for "single payer," government-run, cradle-to-grave health care, must control costs. Waiting two years between mammograms saves dollars but puts women at risk.

The American Cancer Society has compromised itself by recommending, "Women ages forty to forty-four should have the choice to start annual breast cancer screening with mammograms (X-rays of the breast) if they wish to do so. Women age forty-five to fifty-four should get mammograms every year. Women fifty-five and older should switch to mammograms every two years, or can continue yearly screening. Screening should continue as long as a woman is in good health and is expected to live ten more years or longer."

The American College of Obstetricians and Gynecologists continues to recommend the first mammography at age forty, then annually until age seventy-five. Almost all practicing doctors agree with that because we have seen too many young women die unnecessarily when earlier detection could have saved them.

But you should do what your personal doctor tells you!

CHAPTER 2

The Lady Who Couldn't
Find Her Way Home

> *Bodily decay is gloomy in prospect, but*
> *of all human contemplations, the most*
> *abhorrent is body without mind.*
> —Thomas Jefferson

I T WAS DUSK, and the advancing shadows of the tall
eucalyptus trees along the residential street were
beginning to obscure the homes. My elderly neighbor Mrs. Ford was walking hesitantly up to the front
entrance of the home across the street. She glanced at
the two adjacent houses, seemingly uncertain about
which home to enter. From my vantage point, on my
front lawn where I was gathering up my gardening
tools, it became apparent that she was confused as

to which of the somewhat similar residences was the one where she lived. I walked across the quiet street just as she was backing up to the center of the road, apparently to get a better view of all the houses. I said, "Good evening, Mrs. Ford. It's getting rather dark, and it's difficult for anyone to see which house is which, but I believe the one on the right is yours."

Taking her arm, I strolled with her to her door, while engaging her in small talk. She seemed otherwise well oriented, and her conversation was appropriate. She was an eighty-year-old, very cultured lady with a university degree, a rarity in her era. She appeared much younger than her chronologic age. She had lived with her son and daughter-in-law in this home since her husband had passed away about five years earlier. She was still remarkably physically fit and able to walk the mile-long circuit around our neighborhood every evening at a good pace. As I returned home, I was thinking how sad it was that this very bright lady could no longer find her way back. I told myself I must ask her son if she'd been showing any other symptoms of dementia.

This episode reminded me of several other patients with memory loss I had seen in my office over the past few years. Mrs. Brown was one of those, a delightful lady who had always been very self-sufficient and was proud of still having a driver's license at age eighty-five. About two months before, her daughter had remarked, "I'm concerned about my mother. She is getting very absentminded. She repeats the same stories about the same old events over and over.

She has trouble remembering whether or not she has eaten, or what activities she has engaged in just that day or the day before. One minute after a phone call in which she chats with the caller, she can't tell you who called or what their message was! When cooking, she frequently forgets she has things on the stove and burns the food, so I am afraid she might start a fire. When visiting her, the smoke alarm often calls me to dinner. Also, I have noticed her carefully keeping a calendar of the dates of upcoming visits with other family members, doctors, and dentists. She even records the dates that she expects the dry cleaner and the milkman to come, as well as the day that she must pay the paperboy. She never used to need this type of reminder."

Her daughter went on to say that recently her mother had driven to the market and couldn't find her way home. "Luckily, an observant young couple noted her plight. The wife drove Mom home while the husband followed in mom's car."

My receptionist related a humorous but pathetic incident in which Mrs. Brown asked for directions to her regular pharmacy. She left our office and tried to drive there, but came back twice over the next two hours to ask for the same directions. We called her daughter to report these experiences, and the family conspired to have the Department of Motor Vehicles rescind her license and sell her car. On another occasion, she was dropped off at a nearby hospital's imaging department, on time for her appointment. While sitting and waiting for the imaging technician, she left and walked back to her house. She reported later, "I forgot what I was there for, so I went home." She presented again at the same department eight hours later, but after closing time. She told the janitor, "I have an appointment for a CAT scan."

He reportedly replied, "Well, did you bring your cat?" So she walked home again.

I suggested it might be time for a family member to move in with her, or get a part- or full-time caregiver.

Another longtime patient in his early fifties, James, was one of our favorites because he was so happy-go-lucky and always gave staff and other patients in the waiting room a good laugh. Unfortunately, he was a chronic alcoholic with two dementia causes in play, alcohol and Alzheimer's disease. Once his mental status began to deteriorate, it declined rapidly. Within two years of the onset of symptoms, he progressed from forgetfulness and misplacing things, through loss of short- and long-term memory, and through loss of skills and personality changes to severe dementia, ultimately requiring hospitalization. There was an element of comedy in this case on the day his family brought him to the local hospital to be admitted for substance abuse and custodial care. While his daughter was signing the admitting papers, James wandered off. For the next two hours, it was like a Keystone Cops routine as he cleverly eluded the nursing staff and security guards by hiding in restrooms, closets, and storerooms. He was eventually spotted running through an operating room where surgery was in progress and leaving through the emergency exit, leaving the door open and the bell ringing. His pursuers were reluctant to go through the operating room, and the patient escaped out to the parking lot. Many hours later, he was brought back by the police. Reportedly, he had walked up to a private residence several miles from the hospital, knocked on the door, and announced, "I am James White, and I am lost." The homeowner apparently invited him in, because he had heard on the news that the missing patient was harmless. He then called the police to come and get James.

Dementia, in general, is so pervasive that one needn't look far for examples, even at an early age. Ted was a highly regarded aerospace engineer whose work performance gradually deteriorated to the point that his company offered him a comfortable retirement package at age fifty. His wife and family had witnessed the pitiful progression of symptoms similar to those described in the preceding stories. After retirement, his cognitive skills continued to decline, culminating in Ted spending many hours a day in his garage workshop, where his son had removed the extension cords from the power devices so that his father could not hurt himself. Ted did nothing all day but repeatedly rearrange his tools and sweep the floor. Ted's other favorite pastime was leafing through every page of a magazine, reading aloud every single word. His conversations were like a word salad and made no sense. As the years went by he became a terrible burden to his wife. He often wandered away from home in his pajamas and slippers and got lost. The police would find him and bring him home two or three times a week. He gradually became antisocial, agitated, obstreperous, and finally combative. Still, his wife would not give in to pleas from the family and his doctor to place him in a nursing facility with twenty-four-hour care. She said, "He is the light of my life, and I will be with him to the end. I will not dump him into a nursing home! But I could use a part-time caregiver's help with bladder and bowel issues and bathing."

All of these patients had Alzheimer's disease (AD), a type of dementia that accounts for 70 percent of all cases of dementia. It is an insidious, progressive, degenerative disorder of the brain of unknown etiology, or cause. It results in a gradual decline in cognition, and memory. It is irreversible, meaning the changes in the brain cells are permanent and irreparable, rendering them unable to function. It is progressive, meaning the nerve-cell changes and symptoms become worse over time. It is degenerative, meaning the cell structures deteriorate, leading to atrophy or shrinkage of brain tissue.

This condition was first described and named in 1907 by a German physician, Alois Alzheimer. He recognized that this typical situation in the aging population resulted in a loss of the ability to register or record new information, hence the inability to recall recent events. He also noted a loss of long-term memories as brain cells died and were not replaced. Dr. Alzheimer and his contemporaries were not able to find any prevention, cause, or cure for this dreadful affliction, and over a hundred years later, no preventive, healing substance, or cure has been found.

The pharmaceutical field is littered with drug research failures that had been touted as potential cures. The best of them currently in use—memantine and rivastigmine used together, have only slowed mental decline. The cure and reversal agents are still on the distant horizon.

Although the underlying cause of AD is still a mystery, in the past two decades, strides have been made by medical scientists all over the world. With the advent of sophisticated brain scanners and cryo-electron microscopy the biochemical pathologic process that has damaged or killed the neurons (brain cells) in Alzheimer's patients has been elucidated.

In 1998, a Scottish scientist found that an abnormal substance called Tau protein is deposited in plaques in the frontal-parietal areas of AD patients' brains, resulting in tangles of neurofibrils in the spaces between neurons; these tiny fibers invade and destroy the neuron cells. Following this discovery, researchers began testing neurochemicals for their potential to slow, arrest, or reverse this destructive process. Some of these new medications have been approved and are in use, but they are exceedingly expensive, and results have been disappointing. Others are presently in phase three of clinical trials, the process of comparing current treatments to the experimental one.

The director of the Alzheimer's Prevention Clinic at New York-Presbyterian/Weill Cornell

Medicine has said that 99 percent of all clinical drug trials for AD have failed. But on a hopeful note, in February 2018, researchers at the Cleveland Clinic announced they had completely reversed AD in laboratory mice. They reduced the abnormal protein plaque formation by removing an enzyme called beta-secretase 1 from the brains of the little animals that had AD. Other researchers agree the results were promising, and in time, could lead to an effective Alzheimer's treatment in humans. Follow-up clinical trials are now underway.

With a cure for AD still afar, early diagnosis becomes even more critical.

AD progresses through seven distinct stages. I implore my readers to be watchful for the early-stage symptoms:

1. Inability to remember why one has entered a room
2. Misplacing things
3. Inclination to ruminate in the past
4. Writing reminder notes
5. Repetitive questions
6. Poor memory of recent events
7. Trouble with performing familiar tasks
8. Difficulty remembering names of family and friends
9. Difficulty expressing thoughts and finding words
10. Difficulty managing money and paying bills

11. Loss of interest in favorite activities and hobbies
12. Muscle rigidity with slow movements like a sloth

If you observe a loved one, friend, or neighbor exhibiting any of the above, please encourage them to see their family doctor, internist, neurologist, or psychiatrist.

If your suggestion is scoffed at or rejected, try this excellent, simple test. Ask the suspect to draw a circle on a piece of paper. Then tell him or her to draw a clock face in that circle, with the hour numbers in place. (If they need coaxing, put the 12 in for them to get them started.) Most dementia patients will omit numerals or misplace them.

Another good screening test is to ask the individual to name as many fruits (or vegetables) as they can in one minute. Less than ten means an appointment with a physician.

Some forms of dementia are treatable, and it is essential to identify and separate those from Alzheimer's patients, who will eventually decline mentally, become incapable of self-care, lead a vegetative existence, become a financial burden on the family, and ultimately require institutional care. The need for institutionalization occurs an average of eight years from the time of onset of the symptoms.

In evaluating a patient for possible dementia, the physician will make the diagnosis primarily from the clinical history. He or she will try to differentiate AD from the other, sometimes reversible and often curable, forms of dementia, such as depression, acute delirium, head injury, stroke, substance abuse, lead poisoning, and other neurologic and endocrine (hormone) disorders. The doctor will ask questions regarding the onset of the symptoms and whether the onset was slow or abrupt. He or she will also want to know about changes in the ability to perform normal activities of daily living and the duration of any such changes.

A physical examination will be performed, with particular attention to the nervous system. It is usual to find no significant abnormalities in the early stages of AD, but contributing factors such as alcoholism, depression, and substance abuse may be revealed. Laboratory tests will be performed to help reveal contributing factors, and to exclude other diseases that mimic or aggravate AD. Then perhaps a brain scan, the ultimate diagnostic tool, will be performed.

Finally, the doctor will perform the five-minute, universally accepted, Mini-Mental State Exam. It is a one-page form the doctor fills out as he or she asks standard questions designed to grade the status of the dementia patient. It reveals orientation, registration (recording of new information), attention, calculation, recall, and language. A score of 25 to 30 is normal, 20 to 24 is mild dementia, and below 20 is moderate to severe dementia. When readministered at regular intervals, this assessment tool is especially helpful for following the progression of the disease over the years.

In a few years, new screening tests for picking up AD in its earliest stages may become commonplace.

As to the treatment of AD, while there is a common perception by the lay public that Alzheimer's is untreatable, much can be done to slow the progression. The doctor will mention nutrition, daily walking and workouts, reading, crossword puzzles, and other mind-stimulating games, etc.

The physician may prescribe medications for treatment of related conditions such as hypertension, hyperlipidemia, or diabetes if indicated, or for the insomnia, depression, or aggressive behavior that often accompanies dementias. More importantly, your physician may prescribe the AD medications that are thought to be the most effective for slowing cognitive decline, although the retail cost may be prohibitive for some.

Regarding prevention, little is known, but several years ago, a rheumatologist at the University of British Columbia School of Medicine in Vancouver, Canada, observed that his arthritic patients rarely developed AD. They all had been taking anti-inflammatory medications (e.g., Motrin, Naprosyn, Advil, Feldene, or steroids) on a regular basis for years, which seemed to protect them from AD. But a word of caution here, those medications frequently cause stomach ulcers.

Other physicians have observed that patients who regularly take medicines for esophagitis or gastritis (e.g., Zantac, Tagamet, Prilosec) rarely get Alzheimer's.

These anecdotal observations have served as the basis for follow-up studies. Meanwhile, large and small pharmaceutical firms have their scientists formulating and testing new medications based on the latest theories of the cause of AD.

For those families unfortunate enough to have a loved one presently inflicted with this abhorrent disease, the prognosis remains uniformly poor. But we must care for them with a positive attitude, and treat them with patience, love, and affection. Try to make them smile and laugh, every day.

The families of AD patients should rely on their primary-care doctors as their principal resource and patient advocate. Of course, there is an essential role for support groups, too.

For the reader who wishes further information, the National Alzheimer's Association (www.alz.org, 800-272-3900) is the leading voluntary health organization for Alzheimer's care, support, and research.

CHAPTER 3

The Lady Who Was
Afraid Of Birds

A LOUD, PIERCING SHRIEK was heard from the examining room at the end of the hall. Margaret, still
screaming, bolted from the room and collided with
the nurse, who had just escorted her there moments
earlier. After taking the patient's blood pressure, and
asking Margaret her reason for today's visit, the nurse
had left the room, as the patient selected a magazine
to peruse.

We asked her to come into my consultation
room to calm her and allay her fears and find the
cause. "No," she exclaimed. "They are probably just
outside that window too."

The nurse quickly drew the shades as I took
Margaret's hand and tried to talk to her. "What is it,
Margaret? What frightened you so?"

"It's those birds," she blurted out. "Those huge,
black, ugly beasts. I can't stand them." Her eyes were

wide with fear. Her face was pale, her palms were sweaty, and her pulse was rapid. I told my nurse to draw up 5 mg of Valium for injection IV, as a calming agent.

We now understood what had frightened her. Our office was on an upper floor of a tall building with a balcony surrounding each level. Outside the window of each room was a railing above flower boxes. For the past several weeks, I had noticed ravens alighting on the rail and plucking at plants that were going to seed.

Margaret was afraid of the large black birds!

After a short time, Margaret regained her composure sufficiently to relate an incredible tale of a childhood event that was the etiology of her ornithophobia (fear of birds).

When Margaret was very young, her father brought home a canary in a small metal cage. To give his daughter a better look at the bird, he lowered it to her eye level. At that moment, the bird fluttered its wings, which startled Margaret and caused her to recoil backward. She recalled that her father said in seeming disgust, "What are you afraid of? It's only a little bird. It can't hurt you." He then said, "I'll teach you not to be a sissy." He took Margaret into a small bathroom and released the bird from its cage, allowing the bird to fly around the room. The frightened canary alternately hovered around the windowpane in an attempt to find a way out and swooped around the room in a vain effort to seek another way to escape. Several times, it fluttered noisily past little Margaret's head, and once became momentarily caught in her hair. Margaret vividly recalled that she cried and screamed while she tried to protect her head and face with her hands and arms from the frightened bird flying at her from all directions.

From that time on, her dreadful ordeal was indelibly etched in Margaret's memory bank, and she never overcame her fear of birds or anything resembling birds.

All through her childhood and teenage years, Margaret harbored a morbid fear of what many people term "our fine-feathered friends." She studiously avoided situations where birds might be present. At times, she even concocted elaborate excuses to stay away from places such as the civic center with its pigeons; parks with their ducks, swans, and pheasants; and the seashore with its gulls and pelicans. She told us that she could not even bear to gaze at a photograph, painting, or sculpture of a bird.

As an adult, Margaret carried this inordinate fear of birds and her avoidance of them into her marriage and motherhood. Her family understood her bird phobia and made efforts to avoid her exposure to any birds or facsimiles thereof. It was inevitable, however, that Margaret would have a few close encounters with them, no matter what measures she and her family took. When that occurred, her response was almost automatic and identical, and she would scream, avert her eyes, cover, and tremble in fear.

Following the incident in my office that exposed Margaret's secret, an irrational fear, I recommended that she and her husband return to discuss it.

When Margaret and her husband came for their appointment, I told them about another patient of mine who had an inordinate fear of elevators and had not used them for years. Often his elevator phobia, which was a form of claustrophobia, placed him in embarrassing and awkward circumstances if no stairway or escalator was near at hand.

To help this patient overcome his fear of elevators, I referred him to a psychiatrist—a physician with an MD degree plus years of study in psychology—with a subspecialty of treating phobias. He cured my patient with a combination of cognitive psychotherapy sessions and desensitization by repeated exposure to the feared object. Initially, the psychiatrist accompanied the patient to the elevator in his building, pressed the call button, and told the patient "just look in when the door opens, don't go in." After a few repetitions of this procedure, they went in together and then backed out. After several more visits, they went in and went up only one floor. After repeated single-floor trips, the psychiatrist increased the rides to two levels, etc., until a few months later, the patient was able to enter an elevator and go up one level alone.

He was then tasked with parking briefly near any tall building and taking different elevators to increasingly higher levels.

Eventually, the patient overcame his phobia.

Margaret, with her husband's encouragement, accepted a referral to the same psychiatrist, who used a similar methodology to help Margaret. The initial phase consisted of mentioning birds in conversations and asking her to look at photos or paintings of beautifully colored birds. After a few weeks, the psychiatrist instructed Margaret to go to a pet shop near her home. However, before her first visit, her husband was to seek the help of the owner of the shop by moving the bird cages to the rear of the store. In this first phase of her treatment, accompanied by her husband, she was to go to the local mall and stroll down the aisle she had always avoided because the pet store there often had bird cages in the window. For several days, they just walked past that store without stopping. After three or four days, they stopped to look through the pet-store window to watch the puppies and kittens at play. That was repeated frequently, until one day, accompanied by the psychiatrist, Margaret entered the foyer of the pet store and stood in a location where the birds were out of view but their chirping was audible. She was encouraged to watch and enjoy the other animals, of which she had no fear, in the front part of the store.

About a month later she paused calmly, at a distance, in front of a caged parakeet. Two months later, Margaret stood triumphantly, but still somewhat nervously, at a short distance in front of several cages containing a canary, a parakeet, and a Baltimore oriole. Occasionally, the fluttering of their wings would recall her unpleasant childhood experience. But for the first time in her life, Margaret was able to see beauty in these delicate, colorful creatures with their sweet songs.

Ornithophobia, which Margaret had suffered from for so many years, is classified as an anxiety disorder. The American Psychiatric Association's *Diagnostic and Statistical Manual of Mental Disorders (DSM-5)*, a three-inch-thick reference text that lists, classifies, and describes every type of mental illness, has many subclassifications of anxiety disorders including the phobias. That publication defines a phobia as a persistent and irrational fear of a specific object, activity, or situation that results in a compelling desire to avoid the dreaded stimulus. This desire to prevent exposure to the stimulus is often recognized by the victims themselves as abnormal behavior. They see their reactions to the stimulus as excessive and unreasonable in proportion to the actual danger. The text goes on to explain that it is a common to have a rational fear of things such as spiders, snakes, or jungle beasts, but avoiding those has no significant effect on the patient's life. However, if the avoidance behavior is a significant source of distress or interferes with a person's work, love, or play, then the diagnosis of a phobia is warranted. Although Margaret's story also had some features of post-traumatic stress disorder, she certainly qualified for that psychiatric designation of a phobia. In the treatment program itself, severe anxiety recurred at times, triggered in her attempts to master her symptoms by confronting the birds. But with determination, and a great deal of support from family, friends, and the medical profession, her phobia no longer compromises her lifestyle or her activities of daily living.

At this writing, she is able, without undue anxiety, to stroll along a beach or take a walk in the park.

CHAPTER 4

The Girl Who Couldn't
Move A Muscle

I WAS FILLED WITH apprehension and concern as I opened the door to the Intensive Care Unit (ICU) to check on Sarah during my morning hospital rounds. When I had left her bedside in the ICU at eleven the night before, she was motionless as well as unresponsive to any stimulation. It was as if she were dead, despite the healthy color and warmth of her skin. It was difficult for me as her doctor and assistant surgeon to accept the fact that this healthy and fit fourteen-year-old had just undergone a routine surgical procedure that went well, yet she had ended up entirely but temporarily, paralyzed post-op.

As I walked into the cubicle where she lay connected to a respirator machine with a plastic endotracheal tube inserted through her mouth and extending down into her windpipe. I watched and heard each slow, life-sustaining excursion of the piston of the respirator as each cycle of the pump filled her lungs with air and then vented.

The anesthesiologist was still in the room with her, asleep on a gurney (a wheeled stretcher) next to her bed, still wearing his operating room scrub suit. He had been so concerned about Sarah's condition that he had stayed beside her all night to be available for any possible further complication.

The registered nurse (RN) on the morning shift was occupying herself with checking the patient's vital signs (temperature, pulse, blood pressure, respiration rate) and observing the monitoring devices and respirator machine, as well as frequently rolling the girl over to change her position in bed.

I gazed down at Sarah's face, hoping to see some change of facial expression. Instead, it wore the same expressionless, yet peaceful look, present since the previous night's surgery.

But as I touched her hand, her upper eyelids slowly lifted a little, and she weakly squeezed my fingers. She managed a smile, in spite of the adhesive tape across her face holding the tube in her mouth.

Thank God, I thought, *that muscle relaxant medication is finally wearing off.*

It was difficult to believe that it had been less than eighteen hours since Sarah's mother had brought her to my office with severe lower abdominal pain.

In reviewing Sara's chart, I had noted that at birth she been the product of a full-term, unremarkable pregnancy, labor, and delivery, with no congenital disabilities. Her infancy and childhood were unremarkable aside from the usual minor illnesses. She had enjoyed average growth and development. She was an athlete in excellent general health. There was no history of prior surgery or allergic reactions to any medication. Her family history showed that good health and longevity were a common trait. Sarah's mother knew of no familial inherited diseases.

Upon taking the history of the present illness, I learned from Sarah and her mother that earlier that day Sarah had developed periumbilical (surrounding the navel) abdominal pain, which had gradually increased in intensity. By late afternoon, the pain had shifted and localized to the right lower quadrant of her abdomen. Then she began to feel myalgia (aching muscles), ill, and nauseous, with the thought of food being repellent. Her temperature had risen to 103°F. This progression of symptoms was classical for a diagnosis of acute appendicitis.

On physical examination, Sarah exhibited involuntary contraction of her abdominal muscles in response to gentle touching of her abdomen (known as *guarding*), generalized abdominal tenderness to palpation, and exquisite tenderness to palpation of the point midway between the umbilicus or belly button and the right iliac crest (the front of the wing of the hipbone). There was also referred pain to that area when palpating the opposite side. A steady, deep palpation anyplace in her abdomen followed by sudden letup of the pressure brought about severe rebound pain. These signs, combined with marked tenderness on digital rectal examination, confirmed the diagnosis of acute appendicitis.

Blood was drawn for a complete blood count (CBC), and a urine analysis was performed. Subsequently, the lab reported a marked elevation of white blood cells. The segmented type of white cells was increased, and the lymphocyte type was decreased. The urine test was normal. These lab reports further confirmed the diagnosis of acute appendicitis.

I made immediate arrangements for Sarah's admission to the hospital on the surgical floor and told her parents she would probably be undergoing an appendectomy by evening, to remove her infected appendix. I also contacted a skillful general surgeon to evaluate Sarah and, if he concurred, to perform the surgical procedure. I was expected to be the assistant surgeon on the case. The surgeon agreed with my diagnosis and alerted the operating room staff.

While scrubbing for the surgery, I thought to myself how well arrangements were going. In fact, the surgical procedure that followed went without a hitch. The surgeon made a small transverse two-inch incision of the skin just below the "bikini line" on the right. After finding and removing the diseased appendix and then exploring in the abdominal cavity, we sutured together the peritoneum (the tough membrane enveloping all abdominal organs), then closed the abdominal muscle layer. At that point, the surgeon asked me to finish the job and "broke scrub," removing his gloves, mask, and gown, and sat down to write orders for the patient's post-op care, as I was placing fine nylon sutures to close the skin incision. I was pleased with how the wound edges came together in perfect apposition, which meant it would heal with a barely visible scar. With that completed, the nurses bandaged the operation site.

Then the anesthesiologist made a shocking announcement. He had been working behind a drape at the head of the operating table, quietly taking care of Sarah in her unconscious state. "Ladies and gentlemen, I am afraid we have a problem here—a serious one. As you know, we use a general anesthetic gas administered through the endotracheal tube, to induce unconscious so the patient experiences no fear or pain with the surgical procedure. Also, it is customary to run a continuous infusion of succinylcholine to block nerve transmission to all muscles so the patient will not move or jerk while you are working on her."

The anesthesiologist clarified how the succinylcholine works. "Of course, the use of the paralyzing muscle agent prevents contraction of all muscles, including the diaphragm and the accessory muscles of respiration, so it is necessary to use mechanically assisted breathing with an anesthetic machine. Well, as usual, I shut off the succinylcholine drip ten minutes before the anticipated completion of the surgery. By now, this chemical should have cleared from her bloodstream. Yet in this case, it is still active, and she is remaining paralyzed longer than expected."

"Oh my god," said the surgeon. "What do you think is causing that?"

The anesthesiologist responded calmly, "This patient apparently has a rare, genetically determined deficiency of cholinesterase, an enzyme we all have in our blood, which neutralizes the succinylcholine. Luckily, it is always just a relative deficiency."

"Well then," I said, "given extra time she will secrete enough of the enzyme into her circulation to clear the offending substance from her system, right?"

"Yes," he replied. "But there is another little problem. Toward the end of any procedure, we discontinued the anesthetic gas, replacing it with oxygen. Since neuromuscular blockers do not affect consciousness, the patient's brain is now awake and she can hear and think. While I have never encountered this operating room crisis before, I have read about it and studied how to handle such an occurrence."

"Great," the surgeon said. "I am certainly glad to hear that. What is your best guess as to the number of minutes or hours it might take for her to come around?"

"Most likely, two to twelve hours," the anesthesiologist said, "but there have been a few cases in which muscle function did not return for days."

Following a check of her vital signs, he surprised us all by bending over the motionless girl and speaking to her face to face, as if in a conversation. He ignored the fact that her eyes were not open and her face showed no signs of life.

He said, "Sarah, I know you can hear and understand me. You just cannot move a muscle. Don't be afraid. Please trust me. Everything is under control. This is going to end well, and you are going to be just fine. The fact that you are not able to speak or move any part of your body is only temporary. Don't be afraid. You will be able to do these things soon," he continued talking to her with great assurance and confidence. "You are probably trying to wiggle your toes and blink your eyes trying to signal us, but you cannot do these things right now. There is a simple explanation for what is keeping you from doing so. But be assured, in a matter of hours, you will be able to talk and move and walk normally. The reason you are having a problem getting back to movements is this—to prepare you for surgery, we had to give you a medication that paralyzes all skeletal muscles temporarily so that you wouldn't move and jerk during the surgery. The involuntary muscles, such as heart, intestines, and bladder, are not involved. Also, we use an anesthetic gas to put you to sleep during the operation. Well, at the end of your surgery, the anesthetic gas wore off quickly, as it should. The muscle-relaxing medicine, however, is not wearing off as quickly as it should because you apparently inherited a rare genetic trait, in which your body lacks the natural enzyme that is supposed to get rid of the paralyzing chemical. Everybody with this inherited trait has some level of the enzyme, and so, with time, you will get rid of the bad chemical. Meanwhile, I am keeping you attached to this machine that breaths for you.

Also, the nurses will keep you warm and will change your position frequently so you won't hurt at pressure points. I know you can feel pain because the relaxing muscle chemical doesn't affect sensory nerves. If your muscle action does not return in an hour or so, then we will move you carefully onto a gurney and wheel you to the intensive care unit, where you will be in the care of highly skilled nurses who will know how to keep you comfortable and monitor your progress. Of course, I will be there too and will stick with you. In a few more hours, or at least by morning, you will be moving around normally."

We were all relieved, as I am certain the patient was, to hear his reassuring description of the problem and the prognosis. Considering the critical status of my patient, I asked for someone to phone my wife and cancel our plans for the evening while I went out to the waiting room to speak with Sarah's parents, which was going to be a daunting task. As the family physician, it was my responsibility to tell them the bad news, and the better news, about this exceedingly rare complication of anesthesia. I tried my best not to alarm them and endeavored to display as much confidence in the outlook as the anesthesiologist had shown in the operating room.

Afterward, I returned to the patient's side and, along with the other doctors, observed Sarah for about three hours. During that time, we spoke only in a positive, even jocular manner since we knew Sarah was listening. Finally, the decision was made to transfer her to the ICU and put her on a respirator there. The surgeon and I then changed clothes and went to the cafeteria for a cup of coffee where we discussed the case at great length. Afterward, when we went to the ICU to check on Sarah's status, we found that there had been no change. The anesthesiologist said, "Fellows, it's going to be a long night, and there is nothing you can do to help at this point, so you might as well go on home. I'll call you when she regains normal speech and movement, or if any additional complications arise." I then relayed these decisions to the parents. They were then offered the private sitting room adjacent to the ICU, for what could be a long night.

As I was driving home, I couldn't help but think what bad luck it had been for Sarah to have this very rare and hitherto sparsely known genetic defect in her gene pool. Sleep was impossible for me that night. I tried every trick I knew to take my mind off the unfortunate events of the day and evening, but I couldn't suppress my concern for Sarah and the worry her parents must have. I kept replaying the scenes over and over in my mind. I assume I was subconsciously trying to bring about a happier ending to the appendectomy on this young person than what had occurred.

The next day, I was elated when I found that Sarah was beginning to show slight voluntary movements in all different muscle groups. After that brief visit with her, I happily went to my office and spent the morning seeing a full slate of other patients.

During lunchtime, I returned to the ICU and was thrilled to see Sarah sitting up with a big smile on her face, talking to her parents with animation and gesticulations. That made my day! When she saw me, she exclaimed excitedly, "I will never have to use any mind-altering drugs to "trip out," after the scary but exciting experience I just had!" She added, "If I had any doubts about coming out of this alive, they were dispelled when I heard you joke about having to stay in the operating room with me so long you might have to send out for pizza!" We had indeed tried to keep our conversation positive, lighthearted, and even humorous, knowing she could hear and understand.

Then she said, "I did try to signal you by blinking my eyes and wiggling my toes, but I guess they weren't moving."

In the days that followed, all members of Sarah's immediate family were tested for a deficiency of the culprit enzyme, cholinesterase. Her mother was found to be the only one besides Sarah who proved deficient, and was probably a carrier of the defective gene. Arrangements were made for the family to receive genetic counseling by a professor at a nearby medical school. Sarah and her mother were advised to wear MedicAlert bracelets so that if a future need should arise for surgery requiring a general anesthetic, an alternative neuromuscular blocking agent could be used, some of which have antidotes.

Oh, how I wished we could have had an antidote when Sarah couldn't move a muscle!

CHAPTER 5

The Man With A Sixty-Inch Bellyache

P AUL WAS DOING what he had done every morning for the last six months. He baited his fishhook with a piece of raw hamburger, gently dropped his hook and line over the side of his dingy, and finally paid out an additional fifteen feet of line. At age sixty-six, Paul was enjoying his retirement, especially the early-morning hours, when he was alone in his boat on a man-made lake that was stocked with catfish biweekly. Occasionally, he would catch one, but most often, he didn't. Like many anglers, catching fish didn't really matter to him. What was important was the pleasure he derived from launching his boat, rowing slowly out to his favorite fishing cove near the western shore of the lake, setting up his fishing tackle, and then leaning back and watching the ripples on the surface of the water while at the same time enjoying the sunrise over the eastern shore.

As his morning on the lake slipped serenely by, Paul would occasionally temper his hunger by eating a tiny bit of the hamburger he used for bait. Often he would nibble on his piece of raw hamburger, and he would reflect that what he was eating was similar to steak tartare at a fancy buffet.

The one thing that detracted from these idyllic mornings was an increasingly annoying discomfort in his belly. After many weeks of hoping that his intestinal problem would disappear on its own, Paul came to my office for some professional help. In reviewing the history of this illness with me, Paul revealed that his mild generalized abdominal discomfort was accompanied by a slight weakness and intermittent diarrhea.

During my physical examination of Paul, I noted no significant findings beyond a mild tenderness to deep palpation of the lower abdomen. Similarly, my digital (gloved finger) examination of the rectum was unremarkable. Due to the nature and the duration of the symptoms, I ordered a laboratory and imaging workup. This consisted of a complete blood count (CBC), blood-chemistry tests, and urinalysis, as well as an upper GI series (gastrointestinal X-rays), and a barium enema X-ray of the colon. (More recently, these radiographic studies have been supplanted for the most part by endoscopy, visualization of either end of the gastrointestinal system using a fiber-optic scope.)

All of the tests done on Paul proved normal, except the CBC, which indicated the presence of a mild anemia (decreased hemoglobin, the oxygen-carrying component of the blood cells). The blood count also revealed an elevation of a certain type of white blood cell, the eosinophils, which could indicate either an allergy or a parasitic infestation. The next step in my investigation was to pursue a reason for the mild anemia and elevated eosinophil count by studying stool specimens for occult blood (microscopic blood in the feces), ova (eggs), and parasites (adult worms). Even if adult worms are not detected in the stool samples, each species has eggs with a characteristic appearance under the microscope. Paul was given appropriate materials for self-collection of his feces on three separate days. Each stool specimen he brought in was sent to a laboratory for gross and microscopic examination.

When these laboratory studies were returned to me as negative, I was truly perplexed; I decided to pursue another angle. In a follow-up office visit with Paul, I admitted to him that after the costly, uncomfortable, and time-consuming tests, I still did not know the cause of his symptoms. I suggested that he see a gastroenterologist (a specialist in disorders of the esophagus, stomach, gallbladder, pancreas, liver, intestine, colon, and rectum). I prepared and forwarded a cover letter to the gastroenterologist, explaining in detail the full clinical picture and enclosing copies of all reports from the investigation to date.

I did not have any contact with Paul for about a month. When he finally came to see me, I had not yet received any response from the specialist summarizing his evaluation, diagnosis, and any recommended treatment. Paul's first comment when he returned was "Why did you send me to that damn specialist?"

"Well," I replied, "I am familiar with that internist's training and experience, and I believed he was the one who with his skill and training would most likely be able to solve your difficult diagnostic problem."

"Do you know what he gave me to treat my belly pain?" Paul asked. "Valium! He prescribed medicine for my brain instead of medicine for my gut! Then, when I tried to tell that specialist that Valium wasn't the answer, he said that I had a condition called . . . wait a minute, I wrote it down on my notepad . . . a psychophysiologic autonomic and visceral disorder! Come on, doc! That psycho stuff isn't the problem. The problem is in here!" He pointed to his lower abdomen.

Trying to allay Paul's frustration, I replied, "The specialist could be right though, Paul, because there actually is a nerve called the vagus nerve that travels from the hypothalamus (the worry center of the brain) down along each side of the esophagus to the stomach and intestine. When you are under stress or dwell on the problems in your life, you could have a succession of little electrical impulses travel down that nerve and caused what is commonly called irritable bowel syndrome. Apparently, the specialist believed that you were experiencing that stressful condition and, as such, prescribed the Valium, because it usually does help."

"Well, he's wrong," Paul insisted. "It's not here," he said, pointing to his head. "It's here." He again pointed to his lower abdomen.

"All right, Paul," I said. "I believe you. I'll try once again to see if I can come up with the answer."

I then asked him to recline on the examining table and proceeded to palpate his abdomen. I tried to visualize each abdominal organ as I felt it in each particular anatomical location. Once again, I did not find any organ enlargement, masses, or tenderness that could give me a clue to Paul's pain. I decided, possibly as a last resort, to test for parasites again. Because such tests are often so unreliable, doctors never order just one, but rather three at a time, as I had initially. I decided it might be prudent to try again.

Voila! When the stool specimen results returned, one of the tests had unearthed the answer—a tapeworm! The lab test reported the presence of a proglottid (one segment of a tapeworm) in one of the specimens.

Tapeworms are any of the species of parasitic flatworms in a class of worms called Cestodes. Structurally, they consist of a scolex (head) and a long chain of identical segments. The scolex is equipped with hooks, which serve to attach the worm to the lining of the intestine. Suckers are also present on the head, which draw blood and nutrients from the host. A succession of new, immature proglottids are budded off the head. As the tapeworms mature and increase in size, hundreds of these segments form a ribbonlike chain that can grow up to twenty feet long. Toward the end of the chain are mature proglottids containing ripe eggs. The terminal segments break off and pass out of the body with the host's feces. The host may be any vertebrate (animal with a spinal column). When the proglottid packet disintegrates in soil, the eggs develop into minute larval forms that, when eaten by an appropriate intermediate host (such as a cow or a pig), develop in that animal's muscles. Human infestation often occurs when the patient has eaten uncooked or partially cooked meat containing the encysted larval form. Because the proglottids of each genus of tapeworm have a characteristic appearance, identification is relatively easy. The pork tapeworm is called *Taenia solium*, the fish tapeworm has the unlikely name *Diphyllobothrium latum,* and the beef tapeworm is known as *Taenia saginata*. In Paul's case, it was evident that he had ingested larvae of the beef tapeworm from eating the raw hamburger he used for fish bait.

Luckily, for every parasite, there is a pharmacologic agent available for its eradication from humans. Following a special order for the appropriate medication, Paul was treated. A few days later, he came into my office and triumphantly placed a glass jar on the counter containing a coiled-up, off-white, ribbonlike flatworm. The entire worm was there, from scolex all the way down to ripe segments, each one-quarter by three-eighths inch in size. Paul said the worm measured five feet in length.

A key lesson to be learned from this patient's story is to avoid raw or undercooked meat or fish. Such a recommendation may present a major problem for individuals with a preference for sushi. Advocates of sushi should anticipate that the raw seafood—especially farmed salmon—that they consume could contain the fish tapeworm.

Possibly the best lesson to be learned from Paul's experience is that a physician must never forget to listen well to patients' complaints because the patient often has an insight into the problem that can lead to the correct diagnosis.

ADDENDUM: That tapeworm, coiled up in a glass jar full of formaldehyde [with no name on it, of course], was taken to a school by my children over the years for their "show and tell" subject, and they always won the award for the most interesting tale.

CHAPTER 6

The Man Who Would
Be A Woman

W HEN STEVE, A tall, good-looking, regular guy
in his early twenties, arrived at my office right
on time for his appointment, my traditionally raised
receptionist was stunned. His blond hair was cut
long, and he wore an above-the-knee lady's dress, high
heels, eye makeup, lipstick, and fingernail polish. She
initially thought it was a practical joke, but then (not
knowing current definitions), she thought to herself,
I can't believe this. He has become a transvestite. So she
wasn't surprised when Steve announced, "From now
on, I want to be known as Stephanie instead of Steve,
and I would like you to make that official on your
computer patient list and on my medical chart."

I had seen Steve a few times over the years for
minor illnesses, and in those brief visits I had not
picked up on any psychosocial problems, nor had I
noticed any effeminate mannerisms. That day, when

interviewing the patient in my consultation room, I was astounded to hear him say that he believed that he had been given the wrong gender assignment at birth.

He confessed that from early childhood he had known that he was "a woman trapped in a man's body," and "particularly when my body changed at puberty, I found that my body and mind are not of the same sex." He began to cry a little as he said, "I am attracted to the same body in another person that I reject in myself."

Steve described the frustration he had endured while trying to hide these heartfelt feelings from his family, their social circle, classmates, friends, and coworkers. He also admitted that he had recently been associating with transsexuals, or transgenders, as they are now called, and they had convinced him that he was such an individual. He told me he had consulted a psychiatrist whom his new friends had urged him to visit. His visits with this psychiatrist had reinforced his decision to become Stephanie in mind, dress, and behavior, and later in body. Oh my, the mental torture he must have been suffering, to make such a profound change in his life.

Some of the terms describing people with sexual-identity problems, such as homosexual, transvestite, and transsexual, are now considered outdated. For current terminology, the reader should refer to the latest edition of the *Diagnostic and Statistical Manual of Mental Disorders (DSM-5)*. Older editions of this text, only one inch thick, describe a transvestite as "a person with a sexual perversion in which one gets gratification by wearing the clothes and adopting the habits and mannerisms of the opposite sex." In contrast, newer three-inch-thick editions define transsexual or transgender as having "a persistent discomfort and sense of inappropriateness about one's assigned sex" and a "preoccupation . . . with getting rid of one's" genitals.

I soon found that Steve did indeed seem preoccupied with changing his primary reproductive organs and his secondary sex characteristics (breasts, voice, hair growth, fat distribution, etc.) to those of the other sex, to gain a new sexual identity.

Before sex-reassignment surgery, the individual must consult a psychiatrist who, through psychoanalysis, may be able to discern the patient's inner feelings and state of mind about his gender. The psychiatrist must confirm or deny the patient's beliefs before any reputable surgeon will undertake sex-reassignment surgery. This type of procedure, in which the patient's respective male or female genital organs are removed and facsimiles of genitals of the opposite sex are created, is fraught with multiple risks of complications. If the psychiatrist disagrees with the patient, long-term psychotherapy will be offered, to help the individual solve his or her sexual-identity problem in a less radical way.

Once the decision to proceed with the sex-change surgery is finally made, hormone therapy is started, employing estrogen or testosterone derivatives to modify the secondary sex characteristics. In the case of a male undergoing feminization, as would be the case for Steve, breast-augmentation surgery could be performed, as well as electrolysis or epilation of male facial and body hair.

Historically, a notable example of transsexualism was actress and singer Christine Jorgensen, probably the first to gain notoriety for receiving a sex change operation several decades ago. Dr. Renée Richards, an ophthalmologist and highly ranked male college tennis player, became top-rated in the women's professional tennis circuit following sex-change surgery, after a successful lawsuit allowed her to compete. Some lady players, including champion Chris Evert, refused to play against him/her.

More recently, many celebrities, even athletes, including Bruce (now Caitlyn) Jenner, a men's Olympic decathlon gold medalist, have changed their sexual identity permanently, much to the disappointment of fans, and have endured criticism for it.

Before Steve made such a monumental decision, I gave him two heartfelt suggestions:

- Accept my referral to a more conventional psychiatrist for a second opinion.
- Allow me to order a simple DNA test (very expensive, because it was new at the time), to see if he had been genuinely assigned by his maker with the male Y-DNA chromosome or the female X-DNA chromosome and, thus, establish his actual biological sex.

He refused the test but said he might follow up on the referral to the psychiatrist.

Steve returned a year later, with the revelation that he had undergone the year-long psychiatric phase of his sex reassignment, and had recently undergone the next stage, a bilateral orchiectomy (amputation of the testicles), thus removing his principal source of male hormones and his only source of sperm—and sacrificing his ability to father children, should he change his mind in the future.

He then made an unusual request. He stated that he needed to have formal identification verifying that he was female so that he could avoid embarrassment and arrest when using a public women's restroom. He brought an official form from the Department of Motor Vehicles designed for this purpose, on which I had to certify whether his gender identification was male or female, and whether that identification was "complete" or "transitional." I could hardly believe that the state bureaucracy printed a form for this purpose. Because he no longer had testicles, but still had a penis, I checked the squares for "female" and "transitional" and reluctantly signed the form.

Steve had also come to me, his general practice physician, to request my assistance with the next phase of transition, which was to provide him with prescriptions or injections of female hormones on an ongoing basis so that he could acquire some of the real feminine secondary sex characteristics.

I was sorry to say, "I can't help you with that because I have no specialty training in the endocrine or hormone system, so I have no idea which hormones to prescribe, what dosages to give, or what blood levels to maintain." I offered him a referral to an endocrinology specialist, but he said he had no insurance coverage and could not afford to do so, and insisted that I provide this service.

Although I disapproved of this whole procedure, leading as it did to radical, irreversible sex change surgery, I respected the patient's right to make his own decisions. At no cost to my patient, I obtained a telephone consultation as a professional favor with a colleague who was an associate professor of endocrinology at a medical school. With this endocrinologist's guidance as to dosage and administration of the hormones that the patient needed, as well as advice on blood studies to monitor results, my management of his female hormone therapy fulfilled Steve's wish to achieve some physiologic and anatomical changes, including a little breast enlargement and perhaps a change in the register of his voice.

Steve then returned to the unorthodox surgeon who had removed his testicles, for the final act of the sex change drama, the further desecration of the patient's body by amputation of the penis at its base, then creation of a rudimentary vagina and vulva, utilizing the redundant penile and scrotal sac tissues as well as skin grafting.

Approximately three months later, my nurse was on her way home after a late day at the office, when she saw Stephanie. She was one of three women a half block apart, strolling or standing on the curb on a well-traveled street in Olde Towne. All three were wearing very short skirts and tight sweaters over what looked like padded bras. Two of them were talking through an open window to male drivers stopped near the curb. They were apparently soliciting for sex partners.

We had assumed that Stephanie's post-op social and sexual life would be that of typical transgenders, which is dating straight men. Some, however, pose as female prostitutes, trying to make themselves seductively attractive to men in order to engage in sexual activities with the perceived "opposite" sex. Sadly, Stephanie became one of those.

Such encounters presumably must lead to a surprise for their unsuspecting clients. It's common for "street walkers" and their "Johns" to be arrested for this type of activity. We all hoped we would not see her name in our small-town newspaper.

Stephanie later returned to my office for an unrelated medical condition. Outwardly, she appeared to be happy playing her new role. She confided, "I have a steady boyfriend, a fellow employee where I work as a secretary." The boyfriend was apparently unaware of the fact that Stephanie used to be Steve.

CHAPTER 7

The Lady Who Went Deaf Overnight

J EAN WAS A pleasant, cheerful, middle-aged, highly
intelligent woman who worked as an independent
computer programmer and whose skills were in high
demand by local businesses.

She had just awakened from a restful night's
sleep, and as she slowly opened her eyes, she noticed
that the light filtering through the shutters was too
bright for this time of year. Realizing that she had
overslept, she suddenly sat straight up and said, "Oh
hell! I'm late for work!"

She grabbed her old windup clock and found
the alarm, which should have awakened her, had
rung and run right down. Confused, she lay back
down on her pillow and tried to understand what
could have happened. Then she realized that her bedroom was too quiet.

She was used to hearing the children next door playing in their yard before school each morning—but not this morning. Living only a few miles from an air base, she was accustomed to the sound of jets taking off and passing overhead. And more recently, she had also become accustomed to the din of power saws and nail guns as workers remodeled a house across the street. But today, for some reason, all of these sounds were absent.

The only sound Jean heard now was a continuous, low-level but high-pitched ringing or hissing called *tinnitus*. She covered one ear and then the other and discovered that the annoying sound affected both ears equally. As a feeling of anxiety began to sweep over her, a few other tests that should produce audible sounds came to mind. She picked up the telephone and listened for a dial tone, but she couldn't hear it in either ear.

Becoming more frustrated, Jean rolled over to the other side of her bed and turned on her radio, tuning it to the frequency of her favorite morning talk show. She jacked up the volume as far as it would go and heard a noise, but no talking. Then she clapped her hands and did not get the familiar percussion sound. She jumped out of bed, now quite shaken with the frightening realization that something terrible had happened to her hearing overnight.

Trying to think of a reason for her deafness, she reassured herself: *Probably nothing bad is wrong. I'll bet my ears are just plugged by excessive wax.* She recalled that many years ago, she had partially lost her hearing, and upon examination her doctor had noted that excessive amounts of cerumen (earwax) on one side had dampened the vibrations of the tympanic membrane that forms the eardrum. He syringed it out, which fixed it. That thought comforted her now, but only briefly. When Jean flushed the toilet and watched the water spiraling down counterclockwise, but silently, the feeling of fear and panic overwhelmed her again. She stepped over to the sink and turned on the hot and cold water faucets full blast; she saw the water running but heard nothing. Becoming angry, Jean went out into her garden, picked up a nearby potted plant, and smashed it on the pool deck. Although her action resulted in a pot broken into many shards, all she perceived was a distant, low-level noise.

Now at a peak level of frustration, the poor lady screamed as loud as she could, hearing and feeling only a little sound and vibration inside her head. Her worst fears were now confirmed. She blurted out, "My god! I've gone deaf overnight!" She sat down on her bed and cried herself to sleep. After reawakening, she desperately picked up her telephone, but as she prepared to dial my office number, she realized that wouldn't work. Knowing she needed immediate medical attention, and knowing us well enough to be confident that we would see her without an appointment, she dressed hurriedly and got in her car. Although she could not hear the motor start, she felt the vibrations of the engine. Fear gripped her whole being as she drove to my office. She could see the signal lights changing, other cars and trucks moving, and people walking, but all in an eerie silence.

Upon arriving at my office, Jean startled my smiling receptionist with her statement, "I want to see the doctor now, please, it's urgent—I went deaf overnight!" She began to cry, and my receptionist cried too, as she took the poor lady's hand and led her down the hall to me. Then the receptionist brought a large clipboard with a lined pad for me to write down my questions, thoughts, and plans to show the patient.

I began by writing how sorry and sad I was that this dreadful condition had befallen her but that I had seen it before and it might well be temporary. I wrote that although the cause was unknown, a few things could be done to lessen the hearing loss so that at the very least, some hearing would return.

Then I wrote, "Tell me your story."

Meanwhile, we put in a call to a world-renowned otologist—an expert in the field of the ear and diseases affecting the ear—whose office happened to be only a mile away.

It soon became apparent that Jean had suffered a frightening affliction called idiopathic sudden hearing loss. (Idiopathic refers to the absence of a recognizable cause.) I had encountered similar cases several times, but none as severe as what she was now describing.

Since diagnosing this condition would require a good history, I wrote down these questions for Jean to respond to verbally:

"Are both ears involved equally?" (This was crucial information because 90 percent of such cases are unilateral).

"Have you recently been ill with a cold or flu virus, fever, or intestinal problems?"

"Have you been taking any over-the-counter medications that might be ototoxic or neurotoxic, such as many 'health' foods, aspirin, anti-inflammatory medications, or diuretic water pills?"

"Have you recently been treated for cancer with a chemotherapy agent?"

"Are you being treated for any condition by your gynecologist or dermatologist that I am not aware of?"

"Has there been any recent exposure to acoustic trauma, such as loud noises from a gunshot, a jet engine, or a jackhammer?"

"Have you been deep-sea diving or surfing where you could have received a blow to the ears?"

She shook her head and answered no to all of my questions.

Next, I conducted a brief general physical examination to search for evidence of such conditions. I inspected the external auditory canals (ear openings) with an otoscope to view the tympanic membranes (eardrums) but found them to be normal. There was no excessive cerumen present.

I inspected the pharynx at the back of her throat for inflammation and the skin about the ears for any clusters of blisters that might indicate a herpes simplex (cold sore) or herpes zoster (shingles) virus infection.

I used a tuning fork to perform simple tests that if positive would suggest that Jean had a sensori-neural-type hearing loss. This type of hearing deficit is the worst kind because it usually means that the auditory nerve, which senses sound vibrations of the tympanic membrane and transfers the information to the brain, has been severely damaged and could remain so permanently. I was hoping that my patient would have the other type of hearing loss, a mechanical conduction deficit caused by something such as a perforated tympanic membrane or fluid in the middle ear preventing the tympanic membrane from vibrating. Such defects are all easily correctable.

After finishing my workup, I wrote my provisional diagnosis of sensorineural hearing loss, bilateral, severe which I explained to the patient in simple terms. I assured Jean there was hope for improvement with treatment and the passage of time, although I was fibbing a little bit to allay her fear at that time.

Just then, my assistant poked her head in the door and gave us the welcome news that the ear specialist was at his office and would see her at once.

After his initial evaluation, the otologist called me to say that he had treated Jean immediately with high-dose prednisone, a steroid (cortisone-like) medication, to reduce swelling in and about the auditory nerve. Audiogram hearing tests in a soundproof booth had confirmed the diagnosis of near-total deafness. Among other things, he had performed a tympanogram, to rule out fluid in the middle ear, and he arranged for Jean to have the latest-model magnetic resonance imaging (MRI) study of her head, brain, and inner ears. MRI takes multiple slices of X-ray-like but greatly enhanced images of the interior of the body. It is capable of detecting such things as tumors, cerebral hemorrhages, blood clots, fluid collection, and nerve swelling.

In addition to steroids, the otologist prescribed histamine and niacin to help expand the tiniest blood vessels and improve circulation. Although it is not uncommon for an ENT (ear, nose, and throat) specialist to recommend this combination, the treatment has never proved to be very useful. In my experience, if a patient suffers from a moderate to severe sudden hearing loss, there should be significant improvement in one to six months. But if the condition is a total deafness at the outset, as it was in Jean's case, then the prognosis or outlook for the future is very poor.

After his evaluation, the otologist—at that time the only ENT specialist in the county limiting his practice to ear surgery and hearing disorders—reluctantly told Jean in writing, "I am so very sorry, I must tell you that I am stumped as to the cause of your sudden hearing loss. And the treatment of any condition for which the cause is unknown is a just an educated guess. But past trial and error attempts have shown a few medications have helped, so that's what I will offer you. Later, if need be, I can perform a surgical procedure where we implant the latest electronic cochlear device in the hollow mastoid bone behind your ear. It has enabled lifelong deaf patients to hear again!"

He went on to tell her that he expected slow, steady recovery of enough hearing ability so that with the help of the latest high-powered hearing aids and lip-reading she would eventually be able to converse moderately with people considerate enough to speak to her directly, slowly, and with proper diction. Luckily, her occupation was unaffected, as it otherwise would have been in sales or many other lines of work.

This case history occurred just before the invention of the iPhone which would have made two-way conversation easier. But I immediately acquired the latest speech-recognition software program called Dragon Naturally Speaking. After this, when Jean returned to my office for periodic follow-ups, I sat at my computer and spoke into a microphone, and she could look over my shoulder and instantly see my words on the monitor. Later, she was one of the first to get a phone that offered the same voice-to-text function.

Unfortunately, Jean regained only about 10 percent of her hearing. Ultimately, she did receive a cochlear implant, which made her smile again! Presently, years after her devastating hearing loss occurred, Jean wears a pair of sophisticated hearing aids paired with the implant that helped significantly. She has learned to speak in a modulated voice and has mastered sign language as well as lip-reading.

Although this unfortunate incident changed her life profoundly, Jean adapted to it remarkably well. My office staff and I agreed that, outwardly at least, she appeared to have regained her cheerful manner and outgoing personality. I am sure there must be times when she feels frustration, sadness, and even anger at the quirk of fate that deafened her.

We all thanked God that it hadn't happened to her vision instead!

CHAPTER 8

The Sleeper Who Nearly Snored Himself To Death

L UKE, AN AGING judge, felt the familiar sting of the paper clip striking his cheek as he jolted awake. The projectile was fired, as usual, by his bailiff using an elastic band. This nodding off had been happening all too often in recent months. But Luke knew the paper clip was necessary; it had become increasingly difficult for him to stay awake in these deliberations, especially after lunch, even though he had been going to bed early and getting ten to twelve hours of sleep every night. He was well aware that his career and six-figure salary were in jeopardy—not to mention the fact that the lives and fortunes of many others were dependent upon his being alert so that he could make wise decisions. His good friend of many years, the bailiff, had warned him that his nodding off at these hearings was being noticed, and lawyers were talking about it openly. Behind the scenes, there was a movement afoot to offer him early retirement, as he was perceived as being "too old for the job."

Luke's daytime catnaps could occur anytime, anywhere, while he was sitting, standing, or even leaning against a wall. They had begun several years earlier, about the time that he gave up on years of crash dieting and allowed himself to overeat and imbibe too much claret, causing a weight gain of fifty pounds. It was then that he also began to experience night terrors—episodes of suddenly awakening and finding himself sitting up, gasping, and fighting for breath, with his heart pounding rapidly and his brow breaking out in a sweat. These nocturnal events now happened several times a week, each time accompanied by an ominous feeling of impending doom.

His wife, Esther, sleeping next to her noisy bedmate, would awaken and sit up too, to calm him. Each time, he would then lie back down, and soon fall asleep again and resume snoring.

His loving wife of forty years of marriage, Esther was anxious about him, especially when she noticed long pauses between his breaths. She even timed these and found that they sometimes lasted a full minute. From time to time, after an unusually long breathless period, she would poke him in the ribs with her elbow, wondering if he had died and would never take another breath. With that, he would give an explosive snort and partially awaken, and she would tell him, "Turn over on your side. You don't snore in that position."

Having read in the lay press about the condition called sleep apnea, Esther was fearful of having him die in his sleep. She tried to get her husband to visit his doctor about these nocturnal events as well as the afternoon drowsiness that caused him to doze off while on the bench. He always agreed to go, but kept procrastinating about making an appointment.

One morning at breakfast, after a sleepless night, Esther said, "Luke, you haven't been to a doctor for years, yet you know there's something seriously wrong with you. Not only is your judicial career in danger, but your life is also in peril." She began to cry. "I see a red light blinking, and I don't want to lose you."

"Okay," Luke responded, his eyes getting misty. "I'll go."

"This time, let me make an appointment for you with my doctor. He is well trained, experienced, and recently won the Doctor of the Year award because he takes time to listen to his patients' symptoms for clues to the diagnosis."

Esther made the appointment, but Luke later canceled it.

Just as they had feared, Luke was squeezed out of his position on the bench and forced into early retirement against his will, at age sixty, along with the typical golden handshake and a generous pension.

Like all new members of the retirement set, they made the obligatory tour of the Atlantic coast of the United States and Canada to see the beautiful autumn leaves, traveling by bus, boat, and rental car. As might have been anticipated, Luke catnapped several times while driving, but Esther always yelled out just in time to avoid a crash.

After they had arrived back home, Luke worked for a few months, as all retirees do, on deferred maintenance in their home and yard. He painted the house, repaired the fence, landscaped the yard, and created a workshop in the garage. These projects completed, when he wasn't sleeping late or napping, he had nothing to do but tell his wife how to organize her kitchen and run her household. One can guess how that was received. She complained to her daughters, "Your dad is driving me nuts!"

Then one day, Luke happened to develop a red, hot, swollen, sore foot and great toe. It was so painful that he said to his wife, "Take me to your doctor!"

He arrived on crutches, with one foot bare because a stocking hurt too much. After introductions, the patient said, "Doctor, I have never had a pain this severe in my whole life!" Pointing to his big toe, he said, "If a fly were to land on that toe, I wouldn't be able to stand it!"

One glance at the foot was all that any doctor needed to make the diagnosis—acute gouty arthritis—once thought to be a disease of the wealthy. We have all seen cartoons and paintings of kings and nobles sitting with one foot swathed in bandages and propped on a stool while servants bring them bowls of soup and platters of rich, meaty food which we now know are the cause of gout. Meats and other high-protein foods contain purines, substances that raise uric acid levels in the blood and cause gout.

In America, everyone eats like a king, so gout is very common. Fortunately, it can be treated, and resolved in a few days with a low-purine diet and a prescription for Indocin, a nonsteroidal anti-inflammatory drug (NSAID).

In Luke's case, the severe pain in his big toe was a blessing, because it forced him to visit a doctor's office, thus affording his long-suffering spouse an opportunity to disclose her concerns about her snoring bedmate's panicky, breathless nocturnal awakenings.

Between the two of them, they related the classic symptoms of a syndrome called obstructive sleep apnea. The American Medical Association has stated that this is America's number-one invisible disorder, with an estimated twelve million patients suffering chronic sleep deprivation because of it.

Obstructive sleep apnea is an intermittent cessation of breathing that occurs while one is sleeping on one's backside. Caused by airway blockage at the back of the throat, it is due to the soft palate in the roof of the mouth relaxing and hanging down to meet the base of the tongue, which has fallen backward. In this situation, air cannot enter the lungs, and the resulting lack of oxygen in the blood puts the whole body into self-preservation mode, triggering alarm bells. A signal to the tongue makes it wobble which lets in a little air and produces a snoring sound. A stimulus to its sleep center tells the brain to wake up; the chest muscles move deeper and faster, the heart beats rapidly, and the victim wakes up in a panic and sits up, feeling very short of breath.

A few minutes later, the sleeper reclines, and sleep resumes until the cycle is repeated, dozens of times, leading to fragmented sleep, daytime sleepiness, chronic fatigue, and perhaps intellectual deterioration. Sleeping on one's side usually prevents a recurrence, because the tongue dangles sidewise, leaving a small airway.

Obstructive sleep apnea occurs more in men than in women, and most often in those with obesity, as the compression from the extra fat surrounding the neck narrows the airway inside the throat. Any man obese enough to need a shirt collar over size 17 probably has sleep apnea, as well as well as a group of other conditions called metabolic syndrome. This cluster of symptoms includes high blood pressure, high blood sugar, a potbelly, and abnormal cholesterol levels. The syndrome increases a person's risk of early cardiac death.

I arranged for Luke to have an overnight sleep study, or polysomnography, at a local hospital. In this procedure, the patient is hooked up to a variety of devices that record blood pressure, heart rate and rhythm, blood oxygen saturation, eye movements, and leg movements, all under the watchful eye of a technician or nurse, who continuously monitors the devices. The next day following Luke's polysomnography the data was reviewed and interpreted by a physician with a subspecialty in sleep disorders.

When the specialist's report came, we were not surprised to find that he had a severe, life-threatening form of obstructive sleep apnea syndrome. By bringing this to our attention, Luke's wife was probably saving his life. The sleep study revealed eighty-two events per hour, and his blood oxygen saturation levels varied from 68 to 80 percent, instead of the average 90-plus percent. There were 232 oxygen-desaturation events below 90 percent, causing his heart rate to drop to a dangerous low of forty beats per minute on many occasions. There were also a lot of eye movements and restless leg movements.

Due to the severity of the findings observed during the first few hours of the study, during the second half of the night, this patient had been fitted with a continuous positive airway pressure (CPAP) breathing device for the remainder of the sleep study, which alleviated almost all of the signs of airway obstruction.

The consultant's summary of Luke's polysomnograph not only confirmed the diagnosis of severe obstructive sleep apnea but also gave recommendations for treatment.

In some cases, the patient may need nothing more than a dental appliance that advances the jaw and tongue to relieve the airway obstruction. But most will be treated with a CPAP apparatus, which concentrates room air and delivers it by a mask or nasal catheters while the patient sleeps. A few patients such as Luke may require more aggressive treatment such as oral surgery or laser procedure to the back of the mouth, to excise part of the soft palate and the uvula that dangles from it.

When Luke and his wife came to the office to discuss the specialist's report and recommendations, I advised him to obtain a CPAP machine and receive instruction in its use from the supplier's technician. I also suggested that he make lifestyle changes to slowly lose a great deal of weight, perhaps with the help of a dietitian, since his obesity contributed to the throat obstruction.

Later, I referred Luke to an ear, nose, and throat specialist for consideration for surgery as a permanent solution to the problem. But he rejected the surgery because he had become accustomed to sleeping with the transparent plastic mask over his nose and mouth and the whirring sound of the little oxygen-generating machine at his bedside. It had become part of his life. He even traveled with it.

With this regimen in place, Luke no longer suffered from chronic malaise and instead had increased physical and mental energy. He also remained alert all day; his afternoon nap became optional, not mandatory! Even his memory returned to normal, giving him back his old self-confidence.

His wife was pleased to see him become the man that he once was, and thankful that she could sleep undisturbed by his "power mower" snoring.

Soon, Luke's retirement was reversed, and he was back on the bench, enjoying adjudicating cases again.

If you have a spouse like Luke with the following constellation of symptoms, you should insist that he or she see the family doctor or an internal-medicine specialist.

Signs of Obstructive Sleep Apnea

1. Habitual loud snoring with gasping or choking
2. Restless sleep
3. Excessive daytime drowsiness
4. Chronic fatigue
5. Personality changes
6. Obesity, with a shirt collar size greater than 17

CHAPTER 9

The Man Who Could Overheat

J OHN, A YOUNG man in his early twenties, seemed apprehensive and agitated when he arrived at my office for his first-ever appointment. He said he was not ill; his reason for seeing me was the alarming information contained in a registered letter he had received from a stranger. The missive came from a medical school professor in Wisconsin who felt obligated to warn John that he might have a rare hereditary medical condition called malignant hyperthermia (MH). The letter stated that if an individual who had this inherited genetic trait were to undergo any surgical operation requiring standard general anesthetic and a muscle-relaxing medication, he could die of overheating on the operating table!

The medical professor further explained that through his research and daily practice as an anesthesiologist, he had handled some patients who, like John, were carriers of this gene and had experienced life-threatening reactions to inhalation anesthetic gases and muscle-relaxing agents administered to them. Similarly, several other patients who had undergone needed surgery at area hospitals had experienced the same strange reaction to the anesthetic gas and muscle relaxants commonly used for all patients having major surgical procedures. In each case, the core body temperature of those patients soared to uncontrollable, incredible heights, causing or almost causing the patient's death on the operating table.

According to the professor, everyone known to have this rare, inherited condition, now dubbed malignant hyperthermia, must have certain precautions taken before, during, and after every significant surgical procedure.

"So what did the professor say was the connection to you, John?"

John took a deep breath and asked, "Have you ever heard of such a thing as malignant hyperthermia?"

"Yes," I replied, "but in my fifteen years of general medical practice, I have never encountered anyone with it." I further explained to John that during medical school training, one studies not only the prevention, diagnosis, and treatment of common diseases, but also the main features of exceedingly rare conditions. Doctors may practice medicine for a lifetime, and never encounter a patient with such a unique circumstance. However, as responsible physicians, we are expected to maintain an index of suspicion regarding uncommon things when confronted with a puzzling clinical condition.

In the letter, the professor stated that the fatal reaction of a patient with MH had motivated him to do an exhaustive study on it. Because of the gravity of the disease and the potentially life-threatening danger to those who have the genetic trait, he worked with genealogy hobbyists and professional genealogists in the community and with geneticists at his medical facility to begin a search for close relatives of all patients who had died or nearly died of this phenomenon. One of them proved to be a distant cousin of my patient John.

Knowing the condition was due to a mutation in a gene and that carriers of the altered gene passed the mutation from one generation to the next, the doctors were able to put together the family pedigrees of patients identified with the disease. From their research, they found that MH is rare in the population as a whole, but frequently occurs in folks who live in the Midwestern states. This area is largely populated by descendants of immigrants from eastern Europe, especially Czech and Polish immigrants who settled in Wisconsin and Nebraska. These carriers produced many children, a few of whom had the mutant gene in their DNA (deoxyribonucleic acid), the template of all life. The researchers tracked the family trees of the individuals identified with MH on paper and the Internet, using newly available Y-DNA tests to follow the paternal line back five thousand years, and the less-specific Mitochondria-type DNA tests for the maternal line. Of course, many offspring of those immigrants had migrated to other states, as had the family of my new patient John.

John wisely asked whether there was any way to find out if he possessed the defective genetic code.

My advice to him was that he should accept the genealogy evidence! But I promised I would also research my texts and periodic medical journals for other ways to confirm the professor's findings.

Following some investigation, I was able to inform John that I had learned of a simple nonspecific blood test for an enzyme called creatine phosphokinase (CPK), which is almost always significantly elevated in MH patients. CPK is routinely measured as part of a group of blood-chemistry tests on an annual physical exam. Causes of elevated CPK levels in the blood include acute myocardial infarction and liver diseases such as cirrhosis and hepatitis. Also, when muscles are bruised, they release this enzyme into the bloodstream. For example, after a football game, all players usually have a temporary elevation of their CPK.

In addition to this simple, cheap test, we found there was a more expensive muscle-biopsy test available that is conclusive for MH. Initially, I ordered the inexpensive CPK lab test on John's blood. When it showed his CPK was elevated, I then ordered the muscle biopsy, which verified that he was indeed a high-risk candidate for MH. With John's help, we also arranged for his immediate family and close relatives to be tested for this condition.

To allay John's concern, I assured him that he would be safe as long as he wore a MedicAlert bracelet, carried a wallet card explaining his condition, and notified his family and friends about his risk for MH so that he would not undergo surgical procedures without special precautions.

In correspondence with the author of the original letter, we learned more about the inheritance aspects as well as the best pre-op preparations and intra-op cooling measures he had used. Additionally, I held discussions with the anesthesiologists at our local hospital, and they developed a plan and procedures to follow in case John should ever need surgery.

It has been many years since John first came to see me. During that period, John has not required a surgical operation, so he still does not know exactly how his body would respond if he did.

MH was first identified thirty years ago by two Australian physicians. It is related to other pathologic muscle conditions, such as muscular dystrophy and myotonia. The fundamental problem in MH is the excessive body heat that is generated by hypermetabolism of the muscle cells due to sustained muscle contractions. Since almost all of our body's heat results from muscle action, the body feels uncomfortably hot after hard work, and conversely, we shiver to keep warm in cold weather. In MH patients, excessive muscle contraction is apparently triggered by the induction of anesthesia with commonly used anesthetic gases, as well as by a muscle relaxant derived from curare called succinylcholine chloride, which is used in virtually all operative procedures. In addition to abnormal heat production, the sustained muscle contractions require high oxygen consumption and produce excessive carbon dioxide and lactic acid buildup. All of these factors cause muscle-cell damage and could raise bodily temperatures as high as 110°F.

In the past when this occurred, it often proved fatal. But now, in a case when there is an MH reaction, the operating team halts surgery; gives extra oxygen; and administers dantrolene, insulin, and glucose intravenously. Cooling equipment is brought into play. Our local hospital's operating rooms even have a poster on the wall reminding the anesthesiologists, surgeons, and nurses of the sequence of procedures to be followed in dealing with an MH event. As a result, a known MH-susceptible patient, or even a previously unidentified MH patient who develops hyperthermia, will likely survive.

When one considers the thousands of surgical operations that are performed in the United States each year, it is most assuring that only a small fraction of those patients succumbs to this complication. However, MH remains a significant cause of anesthetic deaths in third-world countries, as well as those with socialized medicine, due to budgetary concerns.

Here in the United States of America, with the benefits of the free market and fee-for-service medicine, upon which our health-care delivery system is built, even in rural communities we have no shortage of state-of-the-art operating rooms with high-tech equipment and medications that can handle any operating room crisis. Our anesthesiologists can continuously monitor the surgical patient's heart rate and rhythm, blood pressure, pressure of oxygen, and carbon dioxide level, in addition to jaw-muscle tension, skin color, core body temperature, and other parameters. So those patients known to be at risk of MH or other rare conditions may be given alternative anesthetics, muscle-relaxing agents, and even antidotes when called for.

Readers interested in obtaining further educational information on MH or who are concerned they might have inherited the MH gene should visit the Malignant Hyperthermia Association of the United States (MHAUS) website at https://www.mhaus.org/.

This site offers general information about MH, as well as providing access to the North American Malignant Hyperthermia Registry of MHAUS.

CHAPTER 10

The Lady Who Spoke Gibberish

NAOMI'S FIRST APPOINTMENT at our office was supposedly for a bad cold, but it soon became apparent she had multiple other problems that were much more important and disturbing.

At that time, she was in her early forties, and was a shy but quite personable, somewhat frail, attractive lady with pleasant facial features. She confided in me that she had no close friends who could help her with her problems. She said she had a grown son, whom she rarely saw, and a husband who treated her poorly.

As she began to tell me her life story and reveal her present living situation with her husband, I realized that Naomi was a victim of numerous sad and tragic events that had occurred throughout her life—so much so that she must have been born on Friday the thirteenth with a dark cloud over her head, subsequently broken many mirrors, and had a multitude of black cats crossing her path, causing serial bad-luck episodes!

Naomi suffered from numerous cruel acts inflicted upon her by her husband and others, and had compounded matters by creating an unhappy life for herself with alcoholism. When she first admitted she had a drinking problem, she minimized it. However, my office staff and I had suspected it was the underlying cause of her frequent visits to our office to get treatment for the turned ankle, the sprained wrist, the bruised hip, the banged-up knees, the lacerated lip, and other miscellaneous abrasions associated with drinking and spousal abuse. She confessed that her husband abused her, both verbally and physically. She epitomized the 78 percent of battered women who stay with their abusive husbands and try unsuccessfully to change them. I explained to Naomi that men who batter women might cease their abuse for a brief period in response to a stern warning from a police officer or a judge or even the threat of a divorce, but without ongoing formal counseling help, they never change.

Although it took Naomi years to admit that her husband beat her, she did say earlier that he was having an affair with a younger woman and was quite open about that relationship. He even bragged that his girlfriend had a smaller vagina than she did and suggested that she undergo plastic surgery to make her vagina smaller. My nurse and I were genuinely shocked that Naomi's husband was disgusting enough to make such a request but were more surprised when Naomi asked for a referral to a plastic surgeon skilled in such a procedure. I counseled her strongly against having that surgery and instead referred her to a marriage counselor. We then reported her husband's physical abuse to the county social services department.

Naomi tried in many ways to ingratiate herself with her husband. On one occasion, to make herself younger and more attractive, she applied a commercial wrinkle-remover cream mask to her face. When it was time to remove the caustic material from her face, Naomi had passed out from the drinks she had consumed, and upon awakening several hours later, she was in excruciating pain. Her facial skin had received mostly first- and second-degree burns, with reddening, pain, and swelling of the outer and lower layers of the skin, but the prominences of the nose, cheeks, and chin had third-degree burns penetrating to the deeper tissues. In her confused state, she had also fallen and injured her foot.

When a neighbor brought Naomi to my office, treating her facial burns was paramount. I irrigated the small patches of denuded tissue with a sterile saline solution and debrided the dead skin. To prevent infection, I applied Silvadene cream to those sites and covered them with Telfa nonstick pads.

We then gave attention to her swollen foot. X-rays showed an undisplaced fracture of the fifth metatarsal, the long bone the little toe is connected to. Because the fragments of broken bone remained in alignment, it required no manipulation for reduction, only application of a cast for immobilization. We loaned her crutches and taught her how to use them, cautioning her against weight bearing on that foot until her follow-up visit.

After six weeks, the fracture had healed nicely, but Naomi was not as fortunate in the healing of her facial burns. She had to accept the fact that her disfigured face would improve only slowly over the next year, and the residual scarring might require some plastic surgery after that.

All of Naomi's painful efforts to please her despicable husband proved futile, as he left her for the younger woman anyway.

A year passed before I saw Naomi again for her routine Pap smear and pelvic examination. Before I began the exam she informed me, with some embarrassment, that she had undergone the vaginal tightening procedure. She had looked in the yellow pages and found a surgeon to do the job. On this office visit, she had alcohol on her breath, and once again I coaxed her to let my nurse take her down to the hospital adjacent to our building and introduce her to the charming director of the substance-abuse ward there, but to no avail.

Unlucky things just seemed to happen to Naomi. But for a change, the dark cloud that followed her around finally showed its silver lining. While under the influence on a visit to Las Vegas, she suffered another fall, striking her chest against a hard object and fracturing her sternum or breastbone. When she was brought to the University Medical Center there, the physician on duty noted she was inebriated and took advantage of a law that allows a clinician or the police to take a mentally ill patient into involuntary custody in a hospital or substance-abuse facility for seventy-two hours if they believe the person is a danger to themselves or others. There, the individual is usually confined in a cubicle under continuous view of the nurse's station. The patient's withdrawal phase is carefully observed, and a psychiatrist or physician will prescribe medication as indicated for withdrawal symptoms. After further evaluation by a team of medical doctors, psychiatrists, psychologists, and social workers, that confinement can be extended to two weeks, after which the patient will be released to family or friends and followed up as an outpatient.

At the end of her mandatory confinement, Naomi had begun to fit right in; she stayed voluntarily for several weeks and joined Alcoholics Anonymous. She continued to attend AA meetings regularly, which proved to be the key to turning her life around.

However, one more horrible thing happened to Naomi, and, tragically, she experienced an almost inconceivable case of bad luck and being in the wrong place at the wrong time. She became an innocent victim of an outrageous, evil criminal act.

A neighbor of Naomi's realized that she had not seen Naomi for several days. The neighbor went to her house and looked in the front window. When she saw Naomi on the floor and the room in disarray, she called the police. Upon entering, the police found Naomi unconscious and severely beaten up. After a lengthy period of hospitalization and rehabilitation, she was finally able to return home to try to rebuild her life.

While she was recuperating, the police detectives who were handling her case arrested the two despicable perpetrators, a man and a woman who had broken into her home and victimized her. The police characterized them as "biker types." They had long hair and wore headbands, heavy metallic jewelry bedecking their chests, and leather biker jackets. Naomi said they were unkempt, unwashed, ugly, fat, and vulgar. They acted as animalistic sex fiends. She said that they stayed in her house for at least two days, intermittently beating her and sexually assaulting her. The man raped her on numerous occasions while the woman watched—apparently getting some vicarious pleasure from observing these painful insults.

The full impact of that tragic experience did not become apparent until about a year later when Naomi arrived at my office without an appointment. When the receptionist greeted Naomi, she appeared well outwardly, but in conversation, she responded with unusual buzzing sounds rather than words. Nothing she said made sense. Meeting with Naomi in an examination room, I had to concur with my staff that she indeed was speaking gibberish. The utterances coming from her mouth were not language. There were no real words, just an unusual buzzing and babbling. It was evident that Naomi was unsuccessfully trying to communicate her thoughts. Her gestures, facial expressions, emotions, and speech inflections were ordinary, but the words were not.

Speech impediments, such as aphasia, the inability to formulate words and name objects, are relatively common following a stroke, cerebral hemorrhage, or recent head injury. Naomi's gibberish, on the other hand, was unique. Understandably, she became very frustrated with our inability to comprehend what she was saying. I performed a brief physical examination, with emphasis on the central nervous system (the brain and spinal cord), but found no underlying cause of her speech impediment.

I admitted Naomi to our community hospital and called for consultations by both a neurologist and a psychiatrist. My initial diagnosis was that Naomi had suffered a psychotic breakdown. The psychiatrist arrived first, and following his mental-status exam of Naomi, assured me that her problem was physical, rather than psychological. The neurologist later concurred with the psychiatrist's assessment. A brain scan was then ordered "stat," meaning "now," and the results revealed a subdural hematoma.

When a person receives a severe head injury, two types of intracranial (inside the skull) bleeding may occur. The most common is a subarachnoid hemorrhage, which results from trauma tearing brain tissue or the rupture of a blood vessel, as with an aneurysm (ballooning of an artery), which then pops!. This type of bleeding occurs immediately in a space under a delicate membrane called the arachnoid membrane, which envelopes the brain. The buildup of hydraulic pressure causes severe localized compression of the brain at the site of the bleed. Within one to twenty-four hours of the injury, the onset of a headache, vomiting, or loss of consciousness indicates that the patient has an intracranial hemorrhage. A neurosurgeon is then needed to perform open-brain surgery to decompress the brain and cauterize the bleeding vessels where the scan shows the extravasation to be. The other, less-common intracranial hemorrhage is a subdural hematoma, which takes much longer to reveal itself. It can take a week, a month, or even a year or more following a head injury. In such a case, the head trauma causes a small bleed under the dura, a tough membrane interposed between the arachnoid membrane and the bony surface of the skull. The thousands of tiny blood cells spilled into the subdural space at the time of a head injury are not voluminous enough to cause significant immediate pressure on the brain. Instead, over a period, these blood particles, by their presence, draw fluid into the subdural compartment by osmosis, until enough hydraulic pressure results to cause malfunction of the brain at that location. In Naomi's case, this pool of bloody fluid happened to press upon the anatomic location of the speech center in the lobe of the brain near the temple.

Once the scan confirmed this diagnosis, we summoned a neurosurgeon. Naomi was taken to the operating room, where trephining was performed. The neurosurgeon drilled a small hole in her skull, thus allowing aspiration of the pocket of bloody fluid using a suction device. When the patient regained consciousness post-op, it soon became apparent that the operation was successful. In time, she recovered completely, although as in some other cases, the prolonged pressure on the brain from a delayed diagnosis of subdural hematoma resulted in some residual neurologic problems. Naomi did regain her ability to speak well, but she suffered a minor loss in cognition and recall. She perhaps also experienced a little change in her personality.

After her release from the hospital, Naomi's son, who was now in his early twenties, returned home to care for her. It was gratifying to see how attentive and caring he became after being the "prodigal son" for so long. A few years later, Naomi and her son moved out of state together, and we lost contact with them. I sincerely hope that life has been kinder and gentler to her in the years that have followed.

CHAPTER 11

The Man Who Feared Needles

A S THE AUTOMATIC doors opened to our medical office building, Zack took a step forward, crossed the threshold, and boldly let the doors close behind him. Yes, this time he was in the foyer of the building, unlike a few days earlier, when he could not marshal the courage to go even that far. It was later in the day when Zack had made it up to the third floor by elevator and was sitting nervously in my consultation room that I learned about his struggles in just getting into the building and finally up to my office.

As soon as he was inside the building, Zack began to experience that same adrenaline rush that he had felt in the past with its familiar rapid, pounding heartbeat, sweating, tremor, "butterflies in the stomach with no place to land," and an overall feeling of high anxiety. However, he was aware that this reaction was less severe than previously when faced with being "stuck with a needle." Zack assumed that the difference was due to the tranquilizer medication that I had prescribed for him.

"At least the butterflies seem to be flying in formation," he said.

When Zack had stepped into the elevator, he had begun to experience the usual apprehension. But his fiancée Samantha, who had been at his side since his departure from his home today, put her arm around him and took his hand in hers and gave it a reassuring squeeze. Zack looked at her and said, "I'm so thankful that you're here to help me. You know I wouldn't have made it this far without you."

After exiting the elevator door and entering the doctor's suite, Zack and Samantha were greeted warmly by our receptionist. Zack immediately headed for a chair in the far corner of the waiting room, where he would be out of hearing distance of any medical-type conversation that might occur at the front desk, making him more apprehensive than he already was. He was relieved to see that both the nurse and the receptionist were wearing their personal choice of attire rather than the usual white medical smocks. He'd had a "white coat syndrome" ever since he was a kid. He could recall instances in which he was restrained by white-coated nurses, doctors, and lab technicians while they stuck him with needles or performed other medical procedures on him. But he reminded himself that his fiancée had assured him that this experience would not be like those in his past.

She'd said, "This doctor is different. He has taken care of me ever since I was a little girl, and he has always been gentle, kind, and sympathetic to me. I know they will do this procedure almost painlessly."

Zack thanked her but at the same time was thinking, "I still have time to get out of here," even though he had vowed that he would go through with the procedure today.

A few moments later, my nurse, who was most personable and had a way of putting patients at ease, greeted Zack and Samantha and led them into the back office and to a sunny examining room. Zack glanced around the room, looking for the usual medical paraphernalia—especially the dreaded needles and syringes—but didn't see them. The nurse suggested that he sit next to the woman he loved and wanted to marry. Then, unsurprisingly, Zack blurted out, "If only there weren't this stupid law mandating a premarital blood test, we would have married long ago!" (Although no longer required, at that time premarital blood tests were mandatory in our state.)

Following this outburst, Zack apologized for canceling three previous appointments and being a no-show another time. Seeing that he was embarrassed about the whole thing, the nurse told him, "That's quite all right, the doctor and I understand." She said that the doctor would be right in to see him. "And then," she said, "you'll be out of here in no time saying, 'Gee, there was nothing to that after all!'"

Out in the hallway, I saw that the nurse had put the signal light on, indicating that the patient in that room was ready to be seen. As I was about to enter, my nurse told me, "This is the patient we were expecting who has a morbid fear of needles—so great, in fact, that he has postponed his wedding several times rather than submit to the state-required premarital blood test. He looks like a scared rabbit and may need our extra preparations. His fiancée has given him the Inderal and Valium as you suggested. We brought him straight in, omitting our usual new patient sign in routine."

After entering the room and greeting Zack and Samantha, I explained, "The Inderal tablet you took will blunt the adrenaline rush that you have experienced at times like this, while Valium will help to keep you calm. We plan to numb a small patch on your arm with a little spray such as you have seen sprayed on sprained ankles of athletes injured in a game, who then go back in to play. Then my nurse, who is trained in this and has done it for thousands of our patients, will place the tip of the tiniest needle made through the frozen patch of skin into a vein just below the surface. She will then advance it a little along the lumen, the channel in the center of the vein, will take just a second to draw a little blood with vacuum tubes, and then quickly remove it. It will hurt less than pulling a single hair out of your arm. I will be steadying your arm, and Samantha will be on your other side. Please believe me, this will not be difficult for you at all." Zack seemed quite convinced and said he was willing to give it a try.

We had Zack lie in a supine position, faceup on an exam table, which had been tilted slightly downward toward the head to help prevent fainting.

As we were about to begin, Zack sat up quickly, saying, "Wait, wait!" in a last-minute effort to avoid the perceived ordeal.

But his fiancée put her cheek next to his and gently persuaded him to lie back down. I could feel the muscle tension in his arm and was prepared to restrain it if he should move at an inopportune moment. Zack averted his gaze as the nurse applied a spray of ethyl chloride to the antecubital fossa (the inside of the elbow), followed by wrapping a tourniquet around the upper arm to arrest blood flow and cause the veins to engorge. She deftly palpated the area with her fingertips to locate the best vein, then quickly dipped the tip of a vacuum device with the smallest needle attached through the skin and advanced it to pierce the outer wall of the vein and enter the lumen. She slipped on the first vacuum tube, watching it fill with blood for the mandatory test, and then two more tubes for additional tests that hadn't been done for years, to assess his general health. When the last tube had filled, in a single, uninterrupted motion she released the tourniquet, withdrew the needle, pressed a cotton ball over the puncture site, and taped it down firmly to staunch any subcutaneous bleeding. She also took care not to let Zack see the needle or blood. This whole procedure took less than thirty seconds, but to Zack, it probably seemed like an eternity.

Everyone smiled with relief as Zack sat up and laughed triumphantly.

"We did it! We did it!"

We had Zack lie back down for ten minutes while we monitored his vital signs and observed for shock: hypotension (low blood pressure), bradycardia (slow heart rate), pallor, diaphoresis (profuse sweating) on the upper lip and forehead, or signs of impending vasovagal syncope (fainting). Fortunately, none of these occurred, probably due to the precautions we had taken.

Knowing that Zack had avoided having blood drawn for routine lab tests for years, my nurse had extracted more blood than that required for just the mandatory premarital VDRL test, which screens for syphilis. (Females were required to take an additional blood test to check for immunity to the rubella virus, which causes German measles. If antibodies against this formerly common viral infection were not present, then immunization would be recommended to prevent congenital disabilities in future pregnancies.)

With Zack's permission, comprehensive laboratory studies were performed: a blood count, renal and liver function tests, lipid levels for cholesterol and triglycerides, thyroid, and the hepatitis C test (recommended for all young people who have been sexually active). As expected, Samantha submitted to the mandated tests and a similar battery of lab work without fuss or whimper.

Zack and Samantha left our office smiling broadly, and thanked us sincerely for making his daunting procedure easy.

A few days later, we received a humorous, colorful thank-you card drawn personally by Zack, who was apparently a gifted artist. It depicted the scene in our medical office during the blood-drawing procedure, as perceived by the victim. The sketch included caricatures of all who had been involved in his ordeal. The scene depicted a perspiring Zack bearing a facial expression of fear and pain while being restrained by a larger-than-life, muscle-bound doctor and Samantha, who appeared to have joined forces with his torturers. Our diminutive nurse resembled a Wagnerian Brunhilde, who with a fiendish grin prepared to plunge a gigantic syringe and needle into his arm, which was being choked off by a tight tourniquet. The inscription below the picture read, "Thanks for your patience and kindness, I know now that next time it won't be like this." That card made our day!

Needle phobia is now a recognized psychological abnormality, and is listed in *DSM-5* under the category of blood-injection-injury phobias. The predisposing cause is thought to be an inherited trait. A contributing cause is learned behavior resulting from unpleasant childhood experiences with white-coated medical professionals performing routine immunizations and venipuncture, suturing lacerations, and treating fractured bones.

The severity of the condition ranges from mild anxiety to terror. For some patients, the mere thought of blood, needles, injections, or even just visiting a doctor's or dentist's office or a hospital, is so frightening it results in avoidance behavior that can have a profound effect on the patient's health and longevity. These unfortunate individuals will studiously avoid preventive care such as medical checkups, preventive dental care, immunizations, diagnostic imaging scans, prenatal care, and blood donations. Many will even refuse treatment of serious injuries, or critical surgery, blood transfusions and dental restorations. Some who have this fear will contribute to their early demise through failure to utilize the emergency medical system when they have symptoms such an impending myocardial infarction (heart attack) or transient ischemic attack ("mini stroke") or fail to seek medical help for other conditions such as acute appendicitis, bacteremia (blood poisoning), meningitis, etc.

Patients, such as Zach, who successfully fight their phobias to present themselves for needed medical tests, treatments, etc., will occasionally suffer sudden death from cardiac events during such procedures. These deaths result from what is known as a vasovagal reflex: low blood pressure and slow heart rate induced by an idiosyncratic response of the nervous system to emotional stress, pain, or trauma. While the majority of patients only exhibit vasovagal syncope with these procedures or at the sight of blood, like Doc Martin on TV, a few will have such an abrupt, profound response that death ensues, in spite of precautions and appropriate treatment. In virtually every medical office, at least one patient a day turns pale, says they feel faint, and may fall. The thing to do is lay them down and elevate their legs to shift more blood to their brain.

Needle phobia also has legal consequences, such as medical malpractice suits, defiance of court-ordered blood testing for drugs, alcohol, etc. The refusal of an individual to take a blood test for driving under the influence of alcohol is an admission of guilt and can cause the loss of one's driver's license, the confiscation of his automobile, or incarceration.

Perhaps less critical but yet important are the social implications of blood-injection-injury phobia. Avoidance behavior can affect marriage plans, as in Zack's case; travel abroad requiring immunizations; employment and educational opportunities; and participation in athletic competitions.

Many people unthinkingly joke about this condition, not knowing how profoundly it can change lives—or even end lives!

CHAPTER 12

The Man With The
Hydraulic Penis

J OEY WAS A forty-five-year-old man whose second wife, Fran, was a woman fifteen years younger than him. As in the old popular music song, Franny and Joey were lovers. Oh lordy, how they could love. They swore to be true to each other, just as true as the stars above. He was her man. But his prostate gland went wrong!

Unfortunately, on Joey's annual physical examination, my digital rectal exam revealed prostate enlargement, and lab tests found an abnormal prostate-specific antigen (PSA) test. This simple, inexpensive test is about 80 percent accurate for detecting cancer of the prostate at an early, curable stage. So it is recommended that all men over the age of fifty have a PSA test performed annually.

I referred Joey to a urologist for a follow-up needle biopsy of the gland to confirm the diagnosis.

This type of biopsy is done by inserting into the rectum an ultrasound probe, which displays an image of the adjacent prostate gland on a screen, allowing the urologist to direct a gun at any suspicious-looking islands within the prostate organ. When triggered, the gun fires a hollow needle through the thin wall of the rectum and into the prostate gland just below. When the needle retracts, it contains prostate tissue, which is then smeared on a glass slide, sprayed with sealant, and sent to a pathologist for microscopic examination. In poor Joey's case, the pathologist's report confirmed prostate cancer, a dreadful disease that rarely occurs before age fifty.

We arranged a meeting between Joey, his wife Fran, myself as the family doctor, and a Johns Hopkins trained urologist I had referred them to. We were able to offer only three options:

1. Radical suprapubic prostatectomy.
2. External beam radiation therapy.
3. Do nothing and let the disease take its course. Canadian doctors are told to recommend this option.

The first option, performed at this early stage of the disease, would almost surely result in a permanent cure. But since all sensory and motor nerves related to genital function exit the lower spinal cord and pass through pelvic tissues into and surrounding the prostate gland, post-op erectile dysfunction (ED) is a significant risk of that surgery.

The alternative treatment, radiation therapy, presents a big, ongoing hassle, requiring visits three times a week for two or more months to a radiation facility, where the pelvis is exposed to radiation beams targeting the prostate with minimal damage to the urogenital nerve tracts. This is my customary recommendation, even though it could be less than a lifelong cure.

Joey and his wife chose the more certain long-term cancer cure, surgical excision of the prostate gland and its surrounding capsule. His urologic surgeon was trained in a so-called nerve-sparing version of prostatectomy.

Several weeks after Joey's surgery the couple resumed their sexual activities.

But fate had dealt Joey another lousy card—he was unable to obtain a firm erection, even with the help of Cialis. The desire was still there, but rigidity was not, so vaginal penetration was not possible.

What a blow to the loving couple! But they were not alone in this dreaded, life-changing affliction. About 70 percent of all prostate cancer survivors end up with ED.

Of course, surviving was, and still is, the goal. So Joey and Fran paid the price and now decided to learn to live with it.

Treatment of ED falls into five categories:

1. Pharmacologic (e.g., testosterone, prescription Cialis tabs)

2. A vacuum device used to draw blood force-fully into the penis
3. Self-injection of papaverine medication directly into the penile shaft
4. A surgically implanted penile prosthesis (artificial erection device)
5. Vascular surgery to increase the arterial inflow of blood and restrict the outflow of blood in the veins

Over the next year or so, the couple experimented with the first three of these relatively inexpensive and safe options and found them unhelpful or too complicated or too painful.

Joey decided to go for the ultimate solution—a surgically implanted prosthesis, or erection assistive device. One option was simple surgery for the indwelling type consisting of two silicon rods that are inserted into the two elongated spongy canals in the penis called the corpora cavernosal chambers to replace the blood under pressure that would otherwise be lacking. This implant results in an always-erect penis. When the surgical incision has healed, sexual intercourse is accomplished by bending the rods within the penis forward and upward, making penetration possible. At other times, the still-erect penis is bent downward and sidewise adjacent to the thigh, for concealment by slacks or shorts.

The second option, which Joey chose, was the more complicated hydraulic prosthesis. It is also the most expensive and most invasive, but it would prove to be the most practical and realistic solution for him and his erectile woes, and his wife's enjoyment. In this procedure, the urologist makes three small surgical incisions: one at the base of the penis to insert inflatable silicon cylinders into the corpora cavernosa, another in the lower abdomen to house a small sterile water reservoir and tubing, and the third in the scrotal sac, to install a pump with intake and outflow valves, as well as a little rubber bulb to actuate the pump. Following a three-to-six-week healing period, when an erection is desired, a valve is opened by manipulating it between the thumb and fingertip from outside the scrotum, and then the bulb pump is similarly squeezed, causing fluid to flow from the reservoir into the cylinders in the penis, expanding them fully. It results in a natural-appearing, very rigid erection. When intercourse is completed, reverse of erection is accomplished by manipulating the scrotal valve, allowing the fluid to return to the reservoir, and the organ assumes a natural, near-flaccid appearance and size.

After a suitable healing period, at Joey's final post-op office visit, the urologist instructed both him and Fran on the operation of the valves and pump to allow Joey's penis to distend to its normal erect size, shape, and appearance, and afterward return to its natural state.

After thanking the urologist for restoring to them one of the keys to a long, enjoyable marriage, they immediately departed for their honeymoon suite in an oceanfront hotel, where they could view the sunset and watch for the elusive green flash over the rim of a glass of Dom Pérignon.

The treatment worked so well, they had sexual relations more frequently than before! And they lived happily ever after.

CHAPTER 13

The Men With Pains
In Their Necks

"YOU KNOW, DOC, this pain in the neck is starting to get to me," Jake said. He was sitting erect on a stool in my office while I stood behind him removing a neat row of interrupted nylon sutures (stitches) one at a time, which had been holding together the edges of the healing three-inch linear laceration. I also removed sutures from several other smaller lacerations of the scalp. Multiple tiny facial lacerations were also present, caused by shards of glass from the auto accident he had been in about two weeks earlier.

As I snipped the last suture and eased it out with small forceps, I said, "Everything appears to be healing well on your scalp." I applied the dressings. "Now tell me more about your neck pain, Jake," I said.

He replied, "When I cracked my head open as I went through the windshield, all I could think about was the blood streaming down my face and the terrible pain in the top of my head. At the ER, the doctor and nurses were spending all of their time trying to stop the bleeding, wiping up blood, then stitching up my cuts. At that time, my neck only hurt a little bit, but for the past few days, my neck muscles have become stiff and tight. It hurts so much I can hardly turn my head to look sideways when driving my new Uber car."

Concerned, I said, "Those symptoms can be very significant." I asked him, "Do you have any weakness, tingling, numbness, or pain in your arms or hands?"

"Yes, as a matter of fact," he responded. "I have all of those, especially in my right arm and fingers."

I asked, "Do you know if the emergency room staff took any X-rays of your neck while you were there?"

He replied, "No, I was at the county hospital, and they were too busy that night dealing with other victims of car crashes, stabbings, and shootings. Most of them were injured a lot worse than I was."

This Uber driver willingly took our X-ray request slip and went next door to the radiology department at once. I had requested the standard number of seven views of the cervical spine to rule out an occult, or unde-tected, fracture of a vertebra. My instructions included the note, "Use caution in positioning!" Twenty min-utes later, the radiologist called to report that Jake had a nondisplaced fracture of a cervical vertebra with the bone fragments in anatomical alignment but remain-ing unstable. He had been walking around with a bro-ken neck for over a week! He was fortunate that since the trauma, his activities of daily living had not caused a separation of the fragments at the fracture line. Such movement of the bone fragments could have created a contusion (bruising) or compression of the spinal cord, leading to swelling and loss of nerve communications from the brain to the arms, trunk, and legs, and resulting in quadriplegia (paralysis and lack of sensation and motor function from the neck down). An MRI confirmed this diagnosis and demonstrated that to date, except for swelling, there was no significant injury to the spinal cord itself or to the nerve roots emanating from it. Within the hour, after a quick CT scan, to show more detail, Mr. Lucky was seen by a neurosurgeon, who applied a stabilizing device to his neck and head. This brace consisted of a rigid support rig made of light steel tubing, strapped to both shoulders and chest, and extending up to a crownlike metal band around the top of the head. Four sharply pointed thumb screws in the frame piercing the scalp and partially extending into the skull bones at the four corners immobilized the patient's head and neck. He would be required to wear this awkward, uncomfortable, slightly painful, mechanical rig for two to three months or until the fracture site appeared healed on follow-up X-ray radiographs.

Jake called our office six weeks later to say how good it felt to jettison that rig and to thank us for suspecting and finding his life-threatening occult broken neck.

* * *

Another patient, Joseph, a sixty-seven-year-old, avid cyclist, was riding his ten-speed bike, making a good time along a familiar riverfront bicycle path on a cloudless, brilliantly sunny Saturday morning. He followed the bike trail into the dark shadow of a bridge, which temporarily blinded him, but since he knew the path so well, he continued peddling straight ahead in the dark to the other side of the bridge, where he would emerge into the bright sun, able to see again. However, a moment after he entered the dim area under the bridge, Joe was catapulted over the handlebars, flying through the air upside down and shouting, "Oh shit!"

Joe's next recollection was that of lying on his back in the shade under the bridge, feeling numb all over and not knowing how long he had been lying there. He saw his bike lying a few feet from him, the handlebars askew and the front wheel turned backward, but otherwise apparently not damaged. *What the hell happened?* he asked himself. "I wonder if I'm okay," he said aloud. As he became more lucid, he was afraid to move until he had taken stock of himself and assessed each anatomical part from head to toe. Aside from generalized aches and pains, he could ascertain no localized injury.

Joe sat up, double-checked his limbs for trauma, then rolled over and got to his feet. While standing there, he noticed that he was feeling a little faint and weak. He then looked for and found what had caused his fall. Some foolish prankster had piled up stones in a low, wall-like obstruction across the bicycle path in the shadows. Joe cursed that idiot repeatedly as he kicked and shoved the barrier rocks aside.

Believing that he was lucky to have escaped serious injury, he picked up his bike, straightened the handlebars, and slowly rode home.

That evening, Joe's neck began to stiffen. By bedtime, the stiffness had progressed to pain. He refused to follow his wife's suggestion and go to an emergency room (ER) or urgent care facility but promised her he would see a doctor on Monday morning. Meanwhile, he had a sleepless night and painful weekend. The pain was relieved only a little by aspirin, Tylenol, and Advil.

When Joe came in on Monday, I asked him why he hadn't called my stand-in—or me, since all of my patients have my mobile number. He didn't want to bother me at home. That's what they all say! Following X-rays and CT scan of the cervical region, Joe, too, was found to have a nondisplaced but unstable fracture of a cervical vertebra. He was then referred to the same neurosurgeon who had treated Jake and, unsurprisingly, was fitted with a similar immobilizing neck brace, to avoid displacement of the fragments and injury to the delicate spinal cord. The support by the device relieved Joe's muscle spasm and neck pain significantly.

Joseph's fractured vertebra healed without complication, and approximately two months later the rig was removed. Then, following an extensive reconditioning program, at age sixty-seven he dipped the back wheel of his bicycle into the Pacific Ocean, and six weeks later immersed the front wheel into the Atlantic Ocean. With determination and persistence, he met the challenge of achieving a lifelong personal goal of bicycling across the United States.

* * *

Years later, in the annual lunch-hour touch-football game between the medical doctors and the surgeons on staff at our community hospital, Dr. John Martin, a thirty-five-year-old surgeon, chose the quarterback position. As usual, the game began according to the rules, but quickly deteriorated into a tackle football match, without protective gear.

On one play, after our side had sacked Dr. Martin, he was very slow in getting up. When he finally did get to his feet, I noticed that he was carefully stretching his neck muscles, bending his head first to one side, then the other, then rotating it left and right, and shrugging his shoulders.

When one of the other players asked him if he was okay, he replied that he was fine except for a little stiffness in the neck and slight numbness in one arm and hand. Everyone present advised him to sit out the rest of the game, but he insisted on playing. However, he no longer tried to run or throw a pass, and instead made only hand offs to his teammates after getting the ball from the center. The game ended in a tie, and we all went back to our offices or clinics to care for the afternoon slate of patients.

The next day, I happened to see Dr. Martin as I was getting off the hospital elevator and he was getting on. I asked him how he was doing since his fall during the football game. He said that he noticed that his neck was becoming increasingly stiff and his hand had remained a little numb. As I was encouraging him to get X-rays of his neck, the elevator door closed and ended our conversation.

A week after the game, a colleague walked into the doctor's lounge and said that Dr. Martin was now a patient in the ICU. He had a displaced fracture of a cervical vertebra—in other words, a broken neck—with a spinal cord contusion. The early prognosis was that he could end up with quadriplegia. Apparently, Dr. Martin had been foolishly playing in a softball game the night before and stumbled over first base, causing his second neck trauma of the week. Eyewitnesses to the fall had said that they were surprised at the extent of his injury because the fall seemed so minor. Later, we found out that Dr. Martin did not go for X-rays after the football game, as several other players and I had suggested. Without those X-rays, which could have been done easily on the main floor of his office building, there was no evidence as to just how dangerous the football injury was. So he went and played softball. Considering the severity of his football injury, aggravated by his minor fall at the softball game a week later, my colleagues and I understood what had happened and why he was now in ICU.

Fortunately, the neurosurgeon on call had read of a new procedure to treat spinal injuries. He ordered an immediate, massive, IV dose of prednisone, even before he arrived at the ER. That reduced the edema in and around the spinal cord at the fracture site and later relieved some of the compression of the nerve tracts traveling down the channel to the rest of the body. After the recovery phase, plus an extended period of physical therapy, Dr. Martin regained most of the use of his arms and legs. The physicians and hospital staff were pleasantly surprised three or four months after his accident when Doc Martin walked into the hospital cafeteria with the aid of two canes and served himself a plate of lunch from the buffet. In handling his utensils, there was only a little clumsiness, due to remaining lack of motor and sensory nerve transmission. But all things considered, he had made a miraculous recovery.

Because he never regained dexterity with his hands, Dr. Martin had to give up his surgical practice. He later went to law school and ended up specializing in medical malpractice cases, much to the chagrin of his former colleagues and friends, who consider ambulance-chasing lawyers to be dishonorable bottom-feeders.

* * *

This true story is not about a patient, but is intended to serve as another example of the dire outcome of not following up on occult spinal injuries.

This event happened in Calgary, Alberta, in 1913. I read a story about it in the local newspaper years later when I was in my teens there. Sports historians in Canada and the United States often refer to it, since it is about an American light heavyweight champion prizefighter losing a fight and his life, in the first round, to the Canadian champ, in what the boxing promoter called a world championship bout.

The American champion Luther McCarty, who was raised on a ranch in the southwestern States, arrived in Calgary a week before the scheduled match. He was pleasantly surprised to find that Calgary was considered "cow country," and would provide him with the opportunity to go horseback riding. A few days before the fight, he was thrown from a horse and injured his neck. Being in top physical condition, and thinking that the fall was not too bad, and not wanting to postpone the sold-out match, he foolishly didn't mention the incident to officials.

When the bell rang to start the first round, he was still feeling the impact of his fall from the horse. He cautiously jabbed, bobbed, weaved, ducked, and backpedaled, trying to use his skills as a boxer rather than engage in a slugging match. But halfway through the first round, his opponent caught him with a right hook to the top of his head. Observers reported that the American champ's head flopped around like a rag doll as his limp body fell in a grotesque heap. He went into shock and died there on the canvas. The underlying cause, of course, was being thrown from the horse and incurring an undisplaced fracture of a cervical vertebra, which separated when he was struck on the head, and which in turn crushed or tore his spinal cord. With no rigid skeletal support, the neck muscles were incapable of holding his twelve-pound head in alignment.

The death of the boxing champion was the most tragic of all four incidents related here.

Both of my patients fortuitously survived because they never banged their heads after the initial injury, but Dr. Martin's later fall caused a whiplash that almost resulted in quadriplegia. These true stories serve to illustrate the potential danger inherent in even seemingly mild neck or back trauma. Every hour of the day, every day of the week, in every community, someone sustains a neck injury such as Jake, Joe, Dr. Martin, or Luther McCarty. Critical neck injuries do happen in little league, high school, and college playing fields. They also occur in whiplash injuries from rear-end collisions in traffic, diving into pools, and body surfing in the ocean. Frequently, riders in equestrian events or riding for pleasure suffer severe falls that result in profound neck or back injuries. Work accidents and slips in the home in which one lands in the sitting position often bring about midback spinal fractures. Any person who sustains trauma to the head, neck, or back region, regardless of how minor, should seek an evaluation by a physician as soon as possible. Every parent, spouse, coach, friend, and employer has the responsibility to encourage the victim of an accident to seek immediate medical attention and thereby avoid such tragedies.

CHAPTER 14

The Lady Who Couldn't Stop Pulling Her Hair Out

F OR MANY YEARS, Ruth, her husband, and her children were regular patients of mine. I treated them for the usual illnesses most families have. Ruth, a charming and attractive lady, always dressed to the nines, and appeared to be healthy, happy, and well-adjusted. I was always curious about the wigs she wore, but I was too uncomfortable to mention it for fear it would upset her.

But today, Ruth was here for an earache. Her natural-looking dark blonde wig with hints of gray was of real hair; every curl was in place. As I examined her ear through an otoscope, I had to pull the rim of the ear (pinna) backward and upward to view her eardrum. In the process, the hairpiece slipped upward. That is when I saw her scalp with gray dots and short, stubbly gray hairs of uneven length. She was clearly embarrassed by what had happened and what I must have seen; her cheeks flushed, and I was going to stop there. But Ruth pulled the wig off, saying, "You might as well see it all," and confessed she was forced to wear wigs to conceal her unbreakable habit of plucking out hairs by the roots.

Oh my! How my patient must have been suffering from this self-inflicted deformity. She was mostly bald, a condition known as *alopecia totalis*, as opposed to *alopecia areata*, which involves only patches of skin.

Ruth informed me that in childhood, in order to quell feelings of nervousness, she had formed the unnatural habit of absentmindedly twisting three or four strands of hair around her index finger, applying a small amount of traction, and then finishing the process by jerking the hairs out of her head. As she grew into adulthood, this habit of hair pulling became an obsession with her, progressing until there were no longer enough hairs to pull.

Ruth admitted that she had worn wigs for years, which helped her to keep her problem a secret while enabling her to appear presentable in public. She informed me that her obsession with hair pulling had become so compelling that she could not resist the need to pull out any hair that grew long enough to be twisted around her index finger.

Concerned about the possible damage to her scalp, I asked Ruth for permission to inspect it more carefully. My examination revealed an uneven growth of one-eighth-inch to one-half-inch stubble all over her head, and she had multiple small scars resulting from trauma to the hair roots and occasional follicu-litis (low-grade infection of hair sockets).

Ruth stated that only her immediate family knew about her problem. She had been able to keep her secret because of her adaptability to wearing wigs and her family's support and silence regarding the matter. She'd never felt the need to obtain any psychi-atric or medical advice in dealing with her problem. I wondered, though, why Ruth's devoted husband had not encouraged her to seek mental-health help for her painful and disfiguring habit.

Although Ruth's case may seem unique and rare, it is not an isolated incident. In the medical literature, one can find many similar case histories. Medical textbooks define trichotillomania—from Greek *thrix* (hair) + *tillein* (pull out or pluck) + *mania* (madness)—as a traction alopecia, produced when a patient pulls, plucks, or cuts the hair in a bizarre pattern. The condition is sometimes associated with psychotic disorders, although not necessarily so, and is more commonly found in children than in adults. Occasionally the person afflicted with this problem also plucks out both the eyebrows and eyelashes, as was the case with Ruth.

Apparently, these patients cannot resist the impulse to pull out their hair. The individuals in var-ious case studies state that there is a buildup of ten-sion immediately before the extraction and a sense of gratification during and after the act. Afterward, however, they experience feelings of both sorrow and anger toward themselves. Ruth told me that she had repeatedly vowed not to do it again, but to no avail. An interesting statistical observation is that girls with this disorder outnumber boys by 2.5 to 1.

The syndrome of pulling out one's hair was initially described by a physician in 1889. Since that time, researchers have found that it is associated with a wide variety of other psychiatric disorders—among the most common are obsessive-compulsive disorder, schizophrenia, depression, and bulimia.

In the past, treatment has consisted of psychoanalysis, desensitization therapy, and even aversion therapy utilizing electric shock techniques. In recent years, however, there has been a great deal of success in treating patients with trichotillomania with pharmacologic agents such as fluoxetine (Prozac). These medications are in frequent use for treating depression and obsessive-compulsive disorders in adults. I offered Ruth medicinal treatment to help her overcome this problem, but she declined. Her habit had become so much a part of her existence that she did not see the need to change at this point in her life.

CHAPTER 15

The Man With
Mountain Sickness

MARK, A SIXTY-YEAR old obese, diabetic architect, on a family trip, was enjoying the view from his side window in the small sight-seeing aircraft. It was midsummer, and they had just taken off at the first light of dawn and were climbing to the assigned altitude. The sun's rays were illuminating the pink and orange and yellow clouds resting on the rim of the Grand Canyon below. As the Colorado River snaked its way through the great chasm, the jagged, high, purple cliffs just below the sunrise cast a shadow on the bright canyon floor. Overwhelmed by the beauty before him, Mark thought to himself that he could enjoy it more if he could just breathe more easily.

He had become aware of some difficulty breathing as he and his family were motoring higher and higher into the mountains, and since they had arrived at the hotel a few days before, the shortness of breath and tightness in his chest had been getting slowly worse. He had been somewhat perplexed by how breathless and light-headed he felt as the family were unpacking the car at their little cabin at Bright Angel Lodge on the edge of the canyon. He was even more surprised that he continued to huff and puff after resting awhile in a reclining chair with his feet up. In addition to his breathing problem, he noticed that his feet, ankles, and lower legs had become very swollen during the long car trip, and he recalled that he'd had a gradual onset of a headache as well. He remembered that the previous evening he had developed a juicy-sounding cough, and a wheezing noise emanated from his windpipe while breathing in after a cough or a laugh. Finally falling asleep, he awakened a couple of hours later, still short of breath. He found that by propping himself up with three pillows, he could breathe well enough to go back to sleep.

Now, the droning of the engines and the warmth of the aircraft cabin seemed to be making him drowsy. As he gazed through the reflection of the sun on the window at the beautiful sights below, he was startled to see automobiles and several "weird-looking kids" in the sky adjacent to the aircraft wing. His common sense told him that this was impossible, yet they were there, and he was seeing them. Reluctantly he told his wife Ruth, who was in the seat next to him, about this curious phenomenon. She replied, "You're hallucinating, Mark. Not only that, but your speech is slurred."

Ruth had suspected the day before that something serious was wrong with her husband when she noted that his judgment, thought processes, and memory seemed impaired. Of course, he scoffed at this when she mentioned it to him. She also had been very concerned about his shortness of breath and swelling ankles. Mark rejected her suggestion that they cut the vacation short and go home. Now, Ruth wanted to tell the pilot to turn around, but Mark said breathlessly, "You're getting unnecessarily worried, I'll be just fine. Let's carry on with the flight. We'll be landing in another fifteen minutes or so."

Immediately upon landing, Ruth walked Mark to the car and drove him to a hospital in a nearby community. In the ER, the physician told Mark that he was suffering from oxygen deprivation—also known as mountain sickness or altitude sickness—as well as acute congestive heart failure, with pulmonary edema (fluid exuding into the air cells of the lungs.) He hooked Mark up to oxygen through a nasal catheter tube until his pressure of arterial oxygen in the blood came up from a low of 70 percent to a more normal 94 percent. This reading was monitored using a pulse oximeter (a small electronic device that is snapped onto the fingertip). After reviewing the laboratory tests, the physician gave Mark a diuretic medication to promote rapid excretion of excess water which soon began to relieve his pulmonary edema. He also started Mark on digoxin (digitalis) to increase the force of contraction of the heart muscle, making it a more efficient pump.

Many hours later, and six pounds of water lighter, Mark was discharged with the admonition to leave this 6,800-foot elevation and drive down to sea level as soon as possible.

Ruth took charge. She had her husband back in town and at my office two days later. After reading the ER reports and listening to the story of the week's events, I reviewed his medical history in my chart. It was clear that his lifestyle, about which we'd had many discussions but no success in changing, had set the stage for the altitude sickness. Mark had preexisting morbid, or severe, obesity and advanced chronic obstructive pulmonary disease (COPD) or emphysema caused by smoking two packs of cigarettes a day his entire adult life, as well as inherited hypertension (elevated blood pressure), diabetes, and hyperlipidemia (elevated cholesterol and triglyceride fats in the blood). All of the above had caused fatty deposits in and thickening of his arteries—a condition known as atherosclerosis—and narrowing of the coronary arteries. Poor physical conditioning was another underlying factor.

The ER doctor's diagnosis was a good one in that Mark's hallucinations, dysarthria (garbled speech), and headaches were all due to brain dysfunction called encephalopathy, which was due to hypoxemia (lack of oxygen saturation) in the blood, as well as edema of the brain. Mark's dyspnea (shortness of breath) was precipitated by travel to a high elevation and aggravated by flying to an even higher altitude. The average visitor to the Grand Canyon doesn't have these problems, so it had to be the patient's above-listed multiple medical conditions that were the predisposing causes, plus acute congestive heart failure (CHF) resulting from excess dietary salt and overworked heart. But the main situation was the inability of his little Volkswagen-sized heart engine to keep up with the demands of his Cadillac-sized body.

The CHF resulted in many quarts of excess fluid accumulating in the tissues throughout his body, especially in the lower extremities and lungs, where gravity played a role in his pulmonary edema. He found he had to sit up to keep the fluid in the lowest part of his lungs so he could breathe air in and out of the top of his lungs. What a dreadful feeling that must have been! This assessment had been made by listening to the lungs, as well as by viewing chest X-ray films.

For further treatment of Mark's problems, I pre-scribed oral diuretic tabs to help him jettison remain-ing excess body fluid, as well as potassium tablets to maintain chemical balance. I also prescribed ongoing digoxin to improve the strength of contractions of his little heart muscle.

I referred Mark to a heart specialist and a pul-monologist for ongoing cardiac and respiratory follow-up.

In spite of his health resembling a time bomb ready to blow up, Mark's prognosis or life expectancy could be another decade or two if—but only if—he lost weight, kept his blood pressure and lipids at ideal levels, managed his diabetes well, and quit smoking.

With these factors under control, he could expect to enjoy another decade or two with Ruth and family, and I encouraged him to do so.

As Mark and Ruth left my office, I told him one of the few Latin phrases I remember from my premed Latin course: *Tuum est.* It is up to you!

CHAPTER 16

The Doctor Who Became A Patient

T HIS IS A tale about a doctor who discovered a massive lump in his own abdomen. He knew instantly that a tumor that size in that location was probably malignant. In other words, cancer.

So this is his story. It is my story.

That shocking discovery took place at a beautiful condominium my wife and I had rented on a little island in Hawaii. We had anticipated ten days of rest and rejuvenation of our energy and spirits. On our lanai it was warm, but we always felt the cooling effect of the five-to-eight-mph north equatorial trade winds while enjoying the sea view of passing fishing boats, sailboats, and cruise ships and hearing the waves crash on the lava rock shore below.

My discovery of the growth occurred the first morning of our vacation as I slowly awoke from a deep and restful sleep. I became aware of the cooing of doves and other subtle sounds of this island paradise, as well as the fragrance of plumeria blossoms in the warm, humid air. As I glanced out the wide-open door to the lanai, I saw my wife sipping coffee and working on a crossword puzzle.

I yawned, stretched, and rubbed my tummy. That's when I felt it. "Oh no!" I yelled aloud.

Alarmed, my wife rushed into the room. "What's wrong?" she asked as I continued to palpate my abdomen.

Back in control but unable to disguise my upset, I said, "I just found a huge lump in my belly that doesn't belong there."

As calmly as she could, she asked, her voice quivering, "Well, what do you think it is?"

Without hesitation, I said, "It's a tumor the size of a softball—and that's only the part I can feel. There's no way to know the extent of it."

"Well, what are some other things that it could be?"

"It's cancer until proven otherwise. There is a chance that it could be a benign pancreatic cyst." (As an RN, my wife knew that a pancreatic cyst is a slow fluid accumulation under the membrane covering the pancreas, which slowly balloons up.) "But I know that the majority of masses growing in the abdomen are malignant tumors. They are space-taking, but as they grow they slowly and painlessly push other organs aside and may not become apparent until the cancer is far advanced."

Initially my very human feelings prevailed and, like all my patients to whom I had delivered similar news, a cascade of depressing thoughts occurred. *I don't believe it! Oh God, why me? Why now, at my young age? What did I do to deserve this? What if the tumor has already metastasized and spread to other organs, making it too late for surgery, chemotherapy, or radiation? What if it is terminal? How will my wife and children handle this? How long will I be able to work? Do I have enough investments and life insurance to support my family if I die?*

Within hours these dreadful negative thoughts and feelings of disbelief and anger were supplanted by positive thoughts, logical questions, thoughtful analysis, and diagnostic possibilities. These made me feel hopeful and encouraged me to take action.

I started by being a doctor interviewing me as a patient with my problem.

Me: My chief complaint is I just found a large lump in my belly.

Doc: How long have you had it?

Me: I just noticed it today, but it would probably not have been found three or four months ago, when I weighed twenty-five pounds more. So perhaps it's been there a long time.

Doc: Are there any other symptoms?

Me: No.

Doc: Have you had a previous cancer?

Me: No.

Doc: Is there a family history of cancer? Is there longevity?

Me: No familial cancer found by my genealogy hobby. Longevity, yes. In 1900 the average life expectancy was forty-nine years, but my maternal and paternal ancestors lived into their seventies and eighties in that era.

Doc: On physical exam, no abnormalities found in eyes, ears, nose, throat, cardiac, lungs, other abdominal organs, lymph nodes, skin, joints, or muscles. We could do an X-ray or ultrasound of the abdomen now, but it would be only a little helpful. We need a CAT scan for definitive answers. However, there are no scanners on this island, so you have to go to Honolulu.

Me: But if I go to Honolulu and back for the scan, our vacation time will be all used up! Thanks for your help doctor, but since ten days will not make a difference in the outcome, I shall wait and obtain the scan when we get home.

I told my wife, "I'm not going to think about the tumor or mention it again. Instead, we're going to enjoy our vacation. We'll explore the island, take walks along the beach, swim, snorkel, and sail. We'll drink happy hour mai tais at a waterfront restaurant every sunset and try to see the green flash on the horizon just as the sun sets." My wife agreed to repress her concerns as much as possible. She suggested we go ahead and schedule the scan right then for after our return home, and then forget it and have fun.

That vacation turned out to be a special time together, probably our best holiday ever.

As I walked into our medical building and suite for the first time in ten days, it felt good to be a physician again—the most desirable and enjoyable occupation in the world.

After I shared the highlights of our trip with both my receptionist and nurse, I shocked them by informing them I needed a scan, and why. I had scheduled the study for my lunch hour that very day.

Often, we do not realize how fortunate we are in the United States, having the best high tech equipment and treatment accessible when we need it. In countries such as Canada and most of Europe, which are under government-run socialized medicine, patients are placed on waiting lists for up to a year for scans and surgery, so precious time is lost.

The CAT scan was an interesting experience, not the fearful ordeal reported by many of my patients. The imaging apparatus "slices" the axis of any part of the body horizontally into thin sections, like a ham slicer; takes radiographic (X-ray) photos of each slice; and then enhances the picture quality to show minute details. It then repeats the process vertically. A radiology specialist doctor with expertise in scans views the resulting films. In my case, an abdominal scan was ordered, so it took photos from the diaphragm down to the bladder.

Upon completing the CT scan and returning to my office, I awaited the radiologist's phone call apprehensively.

Finally, my receptionist said, "Doctor, I have the radiologist on the line with your report."

When I took the call, the radiologist said, "Good news. You must go to church regularly because God is taking care of you!" I guessed at his meaning but asked him to explain anyway. "Well," he said, "if I had a mass the size of a football in my abdomen and it turned out to be just a benign cyst, I would surely praise the Lord."

"Yahoo!" I yelled. "Thanks, God!"

My staff came running with big smiles of relief.

Composing myself, I asked the origin of the cyst. The radiologist responded, "It doesn't look like a pancreatic cyst. Instead, it appears to arise from the small intestine. Very possibly you were born with it." That would be an exceedingly rare congenital malformation. It would have to be due to a genetic error, like a gene mutation. He went on to say, "It is most likely a duplication cyst of the small intestine, a rudimentary attempt to form a second small intestine. Or possibly a little bubble that formed under the serosal surface [outer wrapping] of the intestine [sausage casing]. Either way, the cyst filled with fluid and gradually expanded over fifty years until it became large enough for you to notice it."

According to the radiologist, the cystic structure now occupied the entire left half of my abdominal cavity and had displaced all other organs except the left kidney to the opposite side. The only bad news was that the cyst was causing partial obstruction of the left ureter (the tube draining urine from the kidney to the bladder) causing hydronephrosis (back pressure damage) to the kidney.

"It will have to be surgically removed, of course," he told me.

Being well aware of this, I decided to arrange for surgery as soon as possible. I chose a well-trained, experienced trauma surgeon who often handled victims of shootings, stabbings, and work injuries whom I had recommended and assisted for on my own patients needing abdominal operations. He was pleased, and said he was honored that I had asked him. We agreed that the assistant surgeon should be a urologist because of the kidney involvement and the possibility of having to perform some surgical procedure on or about the kidney. I asked for our local Johns Hopkins trained urologist whom I had often assisted on my own patients.

We all discussed the steps needed to prepare for the removal of the cyst.

First, an internist or family practitioner would complete the standard pre-op history and physical exam and lab tests. Following this, I would undergo a small-bowel X-ray series, using liquid barium, to reveal any possible connection between the cyst and the small intestine.

Then the surgeons would review all studies, films, and test results to date to determine the size, shape, and location of the cyst relative to other organs. They would share all the findings with the hospital pathologist to get a second opinion as to whether the cyst was benign or malignant. If she agreed the cyst looked benign, we would postpone its surgical excision four to six weeks to allow for the storing of two units of my own blood, in case a transfusion should become necessary. A significant loss of blood could occur if the cyst was adherent to other organs, necessitating dissecting (cutting) and peeling it away from the other structures. The precaution of storing one's own, or autologous, blood avoids risk of contracting infectious diseases such as AIDS or hepatitis B carried in others' blood.

The urologist suggested that a long, flexible, plastic tube called a stent be inserted through the penis and bladder and up the left ureter all the way to the kidney. This procedure would be performed through a scope under general anesthesia just prior to surgery, so the ureter could be easily felt and identified inside the abdomen and avoid the scalpel.

The surgeon told me that he planned to make his incision from the xiphoid process at the tip of the breastbone down the centerline of the abdomen to the pubic bone, which would provide clear visibility of the cyst and the internal organs. He needed to have full access to the big cyst in order to remove it intact without spilling any of the fluid, which could result in the recurrence of multiple cysts at a later date. He also reminded me that post-op I could expect to have a gnarly, ugly, long incisional scar, "especially since Dr. Brownlee won't be able to help me with suturing the skin closure of the long surgical incision which he has sutured so patiently on other patients that their surgical scars were almost invisible."

Another pre-op precaution the surgeon suggested was a colonoscopy, a transrectal insertion of a long, flexible fiber-optic viewing tube along the length of the colon to note any distortion, partial obstruction, or other involvement of the cyst with the colon.

With all pre-op preparation plans in place, I asked the surgeon for his estimate of my rehabilitation time. He suggested I be off work at least three weeks because of the extent of the surgery. He also insisted that I lose even more excess weight prior to the surgery, so that there would be less chance for complications.

Following the advice I give to my own patients before undergoing surgery, I obtained and signed a durable power of attorney form, designating one family member to make all medical decisions in the event of some complication during surgery or post-op recovery that rendered me unable to make medical decisions for myself. By having such a document, family members are spared the burden of deciding whether or not to use extraordinary means of life support if a catastrophic event occurs.

After arranging for my call group MDs to cover my medical practice, I checked into our community hospital early on the morning of the planned surgery. I became frustrated with the laborious, endless paperwork at the admitting office, but was finally shown to my room, given a gown, and asked to get in bed.

Just before the time scheduled for surgery, an RN came in and gave me the standard pre-op injection of a tranquilizing agent. A short time later, a nurse's aide put me on a gurney for my trip to the operating room, where I was greeted warmly by the operating room nurses and the anesthesiologist—all of whom knew me and some of whom may have voted for me when I won the coveted Doctor of the Year title with over two hundred physicians on the hospital medical staff.

I knew then I was in good hands!

After I was moved from the gurney onto the operating table, the anesthesiologist started an IV by inserting a large-bore needle into a vein and connecting it to plastic tubing from a bottle of sterile IV fluid. As he injected a quick-acting anesthetic agent slowly into the IV tubing, he asked me to count aloud backward from ten.

"Ten, nine, eight, seven . . ."

It seemed like only a few minutes had passed when I heard a soft, gentle, feminine, reassuring voice saying, "Doctor, are you awake? Your surgery is over. You did great!"

I opened my eyes and realized that I was in the recovery room, along with several other patients on gurneys. I was soon impressed with the skill and professionalism of the nurses as they took vital signs and occasionally repositioned me while offering comforting words.

I drifted off and later awakened again. I had my first clear thoughts: *I made it! I'm okay!* And then, *Thank you, God!* I peeked under the huge dressing on my abdomen and saw the zipperlike row of staples that now held me together. Yes, very gnarly-looking.

A little later, back in my own hospital room, I knew that everything had gone well. And there was my wonderful, cute, little wife, holding my hand and smiling. At the foot of the bed were our children, appearing happy, even elated, after what my surgeon had told them.

He had left the operating room to talk to my wife and family in the waiting room and informed them that things had gone well and the team had successfully removed the cyst in its entirety. It was adhered to the surface of the left kidney such that the urologist had to excise part of the capsule off the kidney. The surgeon had discovered a congenital vestigial offshoot of the small intestine called a Meckel's diverticulum which he excised and sutured. The team also performed an incidental appendectomy, to save me any trouble in the future. Gee, that's a lot of surgery!

That afternoon and evening, I was visited by a steady stream of colleagues wishing me well, and even the hospital administrator. I was pleasantly surprised that I was experiencing so little pain after the surgery; however, I did have an annoying plastic nasogastric tube (NG) that had been inserted through one nostril, down the esophagus, and into the stomach with the top end leading to a suction pump. This prevented vomiting of gastric secretions for a couple of days while the bowel remained paralyzed due to anesthetics.

In the early evening, my surgeon dropped by to see how I was doing, as part of his evening hospital rounds. He described in detail his findings and surgical procedures and informed me that the pathologist had already examined a tissue sample of the wall of the cyst under the microscope and had reassured him that it was, in fact, a benign growth, with no evidence of cancer.

As he was about to depart, he told me to use the patient controlled anesthesia (PCA) machine at my bedside liberally so that I wouldn't have to endure any pain and could have a good night's sleep. He stated, "Just because you're a doctor you don't have to appear to be brave in front of the nurses. If you have pain, I want you to press that button. As you know, it will release a measured amount of morphine a limited number of times through the IV into your bloodstream to alleviate your pain." The surgeon reassured my wife that I was doing well and told her she should go home and get a good night's sleep herself.

After they had all departed, the night nurse came in to check me. I told her that the only time I felt bad pain was upon repositioning myself in bed, thus straining my abdominal muscles. So at my surgeon's direction and with her encouragement, I did press the PCA button and took my first injection of the pain-relieving morphine analgesic medication. The reaction was devastating. I was soon overwhelmed with a feeling of nausea, diaphoresis, and weakness. For the next thirty to sixty minutes I lay still, trying to will away the impulse to throw up. The thought of vomiting was especially frightening because the retching could cause surgical incision dehiscence (opening up). While most patients find morphine relaxing and sleep-inducing, I was apparently one of a few with an idiosyncrasy reaction to it. When the nausea finally subsided, I decided to ignore the pain and not accept any pain-relief medicine for the rest of my hospital stay.

I slept very little that night, primarily due to dry mouth and tongue and chapped lips. The RNs came in from time to time, helped me change position a little, lubricated my lips with a soothing moist swab, and gave me a few ice chips to suck.

The next morning, the day shift nurse helped me to get up out of bed, and then assisted me in walking around the room while I held onto and pushed the wheeled IV pole from which hung a plastic bottle of dextrose and water that supplied hydration and sustenance through a vein my arm. This early ambulation was necessary to avoid phlebothrombosis, a blood clot forming in a leg vein, which could result in pulmonary embolism (a piece of clot breaking off and traveling upstream in the venous system, through the heart, and on into the lungs). Patients suffering pulmonary embolism frequently go into shock and often die. It still occurs occasionally today in spite of precautions such as alternating pressure hydraulic leggings to maintain venous return, but was much more common before researchers discovered that the calves of the legs pressing against the operating table or bed for a long period caused venous stasis (slowed or stopped blood flow), allowing blood in the veins to congeal and clot, and setting the stage for embolism. Fortunately, this can be prevented very simply by mobilizing the patient as soon as possible. As an additional protection from phlebothrombosis, I wore thromboembolism deterrent stockings—thigh-high elastic hose worn both night and day while in bed.

By the evening of my second post-op day, the NG tube was removed and I was allowed to have a surgical diet, consisting of broth or Jell-O. On the third post-op day, since I had been successful retaining oral nourishment, the intravenous line was pulled from my arm and I was allowed to have a more advanced diet. Later that day, I walked around all of the hallways in the hospital. When I returned to my room, exhausted, I found that I had been treated specially by the nursing staff. Someone had remade my bed with fresh, crisp, clean sheets and bedspread and opened it back, making it look most inviting.

Following discharge from the hospital at noon on the fourth day, I spent the next few days at home being pampered by another RN—my wife! I gathered strength by walking around our neighborhood with her, holding hands. When I returned to my practice, I found that most of my patients and a few of my colleagues had not even known that I had been away for my first hospitalization, an experience that perhaps made me a better doctor.

The last research on my cyst was done when our hospital's pathologist sent her microscope slides of the tissue taken from the wall of my cyst to her nationally recognized colleague at the university medical school for a second opinion. The report described a benign congenital cyst of the small intestine. It was only the third case of such a cyst reported in the world's medical literature.

CHAPTER 17

Two Men With Claustrophobia

The Fighter Pilot

MATT WAS A captain in the Air Force with more than two thousand hours of flying time in his logbook piloting jet fighters, bombers, and large transport aircraft. He was highly regarded as a "hot shot" pilot by his fellow aviators. He had recently returned to his fighter wing after two years of flying big, multiengine aircraft. One day, a colleague of mine, Dr. Radcliff, who was the flight surgeon at Matt's air base, was offered an opportunity to fly with Matt in the spare seat of an F-14 Tomcat fighter plane, on a demonstration flight. Matt helped the doctor, a nonpilot, squeezed into his cockpit seat and then assisted him with his seat belt and helmet with radio phones. He then provided instruction regarding passenger safety measures, including *touch nothing* on the controls, levers, foot pedals, or switches.

The pilot started the jet engine and taxied to the location specified to perform an engine run-up, accelerating the engine to check and test it. Then they taxied to the main runway, were cleared for a thrilling blastoff, and became airborne quickly. Dr. Radcliff heard the flight controller in the tower order them to proceed straight out and ascend to five thousand feet. But to Dr. Radcliff's surprise, at only 1,500 feet his pilot "turned and burned" to the left, initiating a 180-degree turn back to join the landing pattern.

The controller screamed, "What are you doing? You can't do that!"

Matt replied, "I have a problem and need to make an emergency landing."

The controller immediately changed orders to several other aircraft in the vicinity, then said, "Okay, you are cleared to land!"

They descended steeply and turned left again, and then again onto the final leg of the pattern and land. As soon they were on the ground after a perfect landing, Matt opened the canopy and taxied speedily toward the reserved car parking lot, braked the plane, shut off the jet engine, jumped out, ran to the fence, vaulted over it, ran to his car, and drove off. My perplexed doctor friend was left sitting there alone but managed to extract himself from the aircraft and walk back to the ready room, while mechanics took care of the airplane. This extraordinary event caused quite a stir around the air base, but no one was more surprised than the ace pilot himself!

The next day, Matt showed up early at the flight surgeon's office to apologize to Dr. Radcliff and offer this explanation: "When we were in the preflight briefing room yesterday, I felt strangely uncomfortable and closed in, but dismissed further thought of it until the feeling returned on takeoff and climbing out. Being enclosed in that small cockpit became suddenly unbearable, and I started to panic. I had this overwhelming urge to get out of that little place. I looked at the red button that would blow off the canopy and eject the pilot and seat from the aircraft. I was desperately seeking to do that. If you hadn't been aboard, doctor, I would have ejected and sacrificed a multimillion-dollar aircraft. Although I was mindful of my responsibility for your safety, I came very near to ejecting anyway. I almost left you up there on your own, and you surely would have perished. I fought the urge, although I had my thumb on the button several times but managed to land before sliding open the canopy and escaping."

Dr. Radcliff understood how fear of enclosed places could lead an individual to react as Matt did. He was sympathetic but duty-bound to ground the pilot, pending an investigation. He also arranged a consultation for Matt with the chief psychiatrist of the astronaut training program in the hope that he could help Matt resolve this problem.

The Gunner/Fireman

"Overwhelmed with panic, but restrained by my seat belt, I stared at the red lever just out of my reach that would open the emergency exit window over the wing. I contemplated pulling that lever and pushing that window out to free myself from this sudden, unbearable feeling of being enclosed. Of course, had this been a reality, the aircraft could have gone out of control. Thank God this was something I had conceived in my thoughts only, over and over, but did not put into action. For the remainder of that twenty-minute flight on the little commuter plane, I sat with muscles tense, heart pounding, breathing rapidly, sweating profusely, and trembling, as I continued to fight an intense urge to get out."

I could see my brother Don was still in a state of high anxiety as he related this story to me a few hours afterward at a family reunion. He continued, "I have never experienced claustrophobia before in my life, but this problem began immediately upon boarding the small aircraft. I remember I had to duck down to get through the narrow doorway, and once inside the tiny cabin, in confined quarters, that feeling of being closed in hit me." Upon taking his seat and reluctantly fastening the seat belt, Don listened intently as the flight attendant instructed the passengers in the rows with emergency exits on how to release the lever and take out the escape window. He recalled, "After we taxied to the runway and as the takeoff run was underway, all I could think of was, 'I've got to get out of here, and I don't care how.'" He said, "At no time was I worried about the aircraft crashing. My fear was not a fear of flying! It was a discomfort from being enclosed in that tight space."

Don remembered his wife, who was sitting across the aisle from him, saying, "Don, you're trembling and restless, are you having a heart attack?"

He blurted out, "No, I am not. I'll be okay." He was unable to explain to her what was happening. He restrained her from calling the steward because he just wanted to sit there and try to suppress that terrible feeling.

On the second leg of their journey, Don and his wife were on a much larger aircraft. Yet, although it was less severe, the same feeling of being closed in recurred. He was always in escape mode. Don mused how ironic it was that as a Navy gunner in World War II, he had been confined in small spaces—even inside small gun turrets—without ever experiencing a sense of claustrophobia. More importantly, in his twenty-five years as a firefighter at both a naval base and a commercial airport, his job often entailed crawling into narrow, sometimes smoke-filled, passageways or entering small cargo bays. Not once during these experiences had he even thought about a need to escape. But today, on the same commuter plane that he had flown on dozens of times to get on and off the island where his family lived, he'd had this surprising and unwarranted reaction.

Don's telling of this tale a few times to different relatives at this family gathering acted as a catharsis.

After a few drinks, he gradually became his old jovial self.

A few days later, however, when it was time to fly back home, he confessed that he was becoming apprehensive about the return flight. He had been unsuccessful in securing reservations for alternate transportation by train, and two thousand miles seemed too far to rent a car and drive. Since my physician's license was invalid out of state, we managed to borrow enough of two types of prescription medications from others present to alleviate his claustrophobia. I suggested he take two tranquilizer tablets an hour before each flight, as well as one beta-blocker tablet. (Beta blockers are used to treat high blood pressure, but have the beneficial side effect of blunting the adrenalin rush that occurs when being threatened.) As we said our goodbyes at the airport, I reassured them that these precautions would give him a peaceful trip home.

Don phoned me immediately upon his arrival home to tell me they had made it safely without incident because he slept all the way on the flight! Then they took a slow ferry to the island, instead of the commuter plane. He then told me emphatically, "I can honestly say that my initial claustrophobic episode was the worst experience of my life."

Later, I received a letter from Don confessing that he had experienced an additional claustrophobic episode when the elevator door in the apartment complex where they had lived for ten years did not open immediately one day. That triggered the same panicky feeling, and since then he has been using the stairway exclusively because he is fearful that the door may not open again one day. I praised him for his choice of the stairs because of the benefits of the aerobic exercise involved. I also advised him to make an appointment with a local psychiatrist for his new problem, with a view toward treatment rather than vowing never to fly or use an elevator again.

These two case histories are illustrative of claustrophobia, just one of many phobias. The psychiatric term *phobia* stems from Phobos, the Greek god of fear. Phobias fall into two main categories: social phobias, such as fear of public speaking or agoraphobia (fear of crowded places,) and simple phobias, such as claustrophobia, acrophobia (fear of heights), or zoophobia (fear of certain animals). The symptoms of all phobias are the same: anxiety, intense dread, even terror, all leading to physical signs such as hyperventilation (fast breathing), rapid heart rate, sweating, and tremor. The etiology of most phobias is unknown, but some are known to be a reaction to a single emotionally traumatic preceding event. Such an event can lead to a lifelong fear of the object or situation that incited the phobia. The individual will always make strenuous efforts to avoid these settings. Although the condition tends to be chronic, it can be treated and sometimes overcome through desensitization therapy: gradual, repetitive, positive contact with the fear-arousing stimulus, as exemplified in the earlier story of the woman with the morbid fear of birds.

For Don, desensitization proved helpful, and he was able to ride elevators and fly on wide-bodied aircraft in comfort again. He continues to avoid commuter planes, however, by taking large ferry boats to and from the mainland.

In the case of Matt the pilot, desensitization was impractical for safety reasons, and as such he was never allowed to pilot an aircraft again.

The Girl Who Awakened Paralyzed

W HEN MARY'S WINDUP alarm clock jangled, sig-
naling that it was time to get up and prepare
for school, she awakened from what seemed like a
routine and uneventful good night's sleep. But when
she attempted to get out of bed and stand up, her
legs collapsed from under her and dropped her to the
floor! After struggling to get back to her feet by pulling herself back up onto the bed with her arms, and
falling many times, she discovered that if she locked
her weak legs in a backward position, she could stand
and then shuffle forward. Mary hoped to struggle to
her mother's bedroom in this fashion, pulling herself
from one piece of furniture to the next. However, as
she was reaching out to grab hold of a chair for support, she realized that her arms and hands were also
a little weak, and she collapsed again onto the floor.
Finally, after falling several more times, she panicked

and screamed, "Mom, I can't walk! Mom, I'm paralyzed! Help me! Help me!"

Mary's mother instantly came running to help, and then sat on the floor next to her, listening to her daughter's tearful and bewildered description of how she had fallen when she got out of bed and how the falling continued each time she took a step. She described how she had tried to grasp onto furniture to support herself but couldn't hold on because of the weakness in her hands and arms. She said that she felt a strange tingling sensation and numbness in her hands and feet as well. Overwhelmed by her daughter's distress and weakness and wondering what could have caused it, Mary's mother got her up, calmed her, dressed her, and then arm in arm, with Mary locking her legs for each step, they managed to get Mary to their car. Mary's mother immediately drove to my office for help.

Glancing out the office window at the patient parking area, our receptionist noticed Mary and her mother struggling out of their car and rushed out to assist them. As they entered our waiting room, Mary was walking erect with a boardlike gait, legs hyperextended at the knees. She had to depend on her mother and the nurse for support and balance.

I observed this pitiful scene while speaking with another patient in the hallway, and I thought, *My god, has this poor girl been in an accident or what?*

The nurse and I assisted the girl into the examining room, supporting her on each side.

Knowing this was going to be a diagnostic challenge, I reviewed the patient's past health history in her chart. Until that day, Mary had experienced normal birth and infancy, average growth and development, had never been seriously ill, her immunizations were current and had undergone no significant trauma or surgical operations. Taking a careful history of this present illness and performing a detailed physical and neurologic exam was going to be vital to discovering what had happened to Mary overnight.

I asked if there had been any prodromal, or earlier, warning signs or symptoms prior to this morning. She stated that she'd had a "bad cold" the week before, which had later developed into a flulike illness with fever, malaise, and aching muscles and joints, as well as a headache. She was just beginning to feel better when this partial paralysis occurred. Next came a review of each organ system, during which I asked her about every part of her body. I then proceeded with the physical examination, taking her temperature, blood pressure, and respiration, followed by viewing her skin for a rash or other lesions. Examining her eyes, ears, nose, and throat for inflammation, and listening to her lungs and heart for adventitious or unusual sounds, came next. I then palpated her abdomen for organ enlargement or abnormal tenderness, and found nothing unusual. But, on examination of her neuromuscular system, there was lack of muscle tone and strength from the shoulders downward. A grip-strength meter demonstrated marked weakness of the flexor muscles of both hands. There was also a weakness of extension (straightening) of the fingers, as well as paresis (weakness) of all muscle groups of the shoulders, forearms, and paraspinal muscles of her back.

The most alarming discovery was the nearly total paralysis of all of the muscles of both lower extremities, as well as the absence of deep tendon reflexes when tapping the knee and ankle tendons with the reflex hammer. Mary also had diminished sensation to light touch, pinprick, pain stimuli, and vibration sensation, as checked with a tuning fork in both legs and feet.

Based on the history of the present illness, system review, and physical examination, I concluded that Mary was afflicted with an inflammatory disease, probably viral, of her spinal cord, which involved many nerve tracts responsible for sensation and motor function in the upper and lower extremities.

Physicians such as I, in active practice for many years, will recall treating patients with poliomyelitis, which had a similar presentation, until doctors Salk and Sabin's vaccines eliminated that scourge. Occasionally, we still come across phenomena like Mary's, with a sudden onset of paralysis, seemingly without warning. The one most frequently seen is Guillain-Barré syndrome. It follows a viral respiratory infection or, less often, a gastrointestinal (stomach, intestine, and colon) virus, leading to viremia (viruses in the blood). These microorganisms can invade the spinal fluid in the central nervous system, causing inflammation that results in paralysis that is most often transient, but sometimes permanent. This syndrome or collection of symptoms was named after two French physicians who first described the condition in the medical literature about a hundred years ago.

With Mary's particular pattern of symptoms, Guillain-Barré syndrome was my provisional diagnosis. I assured both Mary and her mother that most patients, after a plateau period, followed by a rapid improvement, and with physical therapy, recover most and frequently all of their neuromuscular functions. We arranged for Mary to be admitted to our local children's hospital, under the care of a competent neurologist in whom I had a great deal of confidence. Her evaluation and diagnostic workup would include a spinal tap, in which fluid from the lower spinal canal is aspirated with a needle for analysis.

The neurologist examined Mary, performed the spinal tap, reviewed other test results, and confirmed my diagnosis of Guillain-Barré syndrome.

Following prolonged rehabilitation therapy, Mary recovered all of her muscle strength and sensory nerve function. She was one of the lucky ones, with a full recovery. She was able to return to all of her former social and athletic activities. She missed a semester of high school during her illness and prolonged recovery, but by taking a correspondence course while in the hospital was able to complete her high school education.

Some years later, Mary married and had children, without any complications from her neuro-muscular disorder.

As a family physician, it was personally gratifying to be able to care for patients like Mary many times. Often the initial prognosis looked dismal, but with the human body's ability to repair itself, given a chance by modern medicine, and with the power of positive thinking and prayer, I witnessed many happy endings.

The twentieth century was a great time to be a physician, when the triumph of science over disease doubled human life expectancy.

CHAPTER 19

The Youths Who Behaved Bizarrely

> *"Let me be mad, then, by all means! mad with the madness of Absinthe, the wildest, most luxurious madness in the world! Vive la folie! Vive l'amour! Vive l'animalisme! Vive le Diable!"*
>
> —Marie Corelli

T HIS TALE IS about a gang of revelers who drank too much, partied and danced too much, and then showed crazy behavior upon returning from Senor Juan's infamous cantina, located at a coastal cruise ship stop.

Senor Juan's is a well-known destination providing wild entertainment for young cruise ship passengers. All who have enjoyed an evening at Senor Juan's must have later told their friends stateside. The word is out that they had the time of their lives there. A "mind-blowing, out-of-body experience" is the usual phrase used to describe an evening at Senor Juan's.

For a very brief time in my medical career, I was a cruise ship doctor. Having had an opportunity to substitute for the ship's regular physician, I signed on for a luxury cruise for two, with modest pay, for two weeks. Although I had two years' experience as an ER physician, it was a daunting assignment. Serving as the only ship's doctor and being responsible for the medical needs and lives of one thousand passengers and three hundred crew, with the help of only one assistant, an RN, would be a challenge. It would be especially difficult to decide if a critically-ill patient might need to be taken ashore by helicopter, at a flat rate of $10,000.

As if that wasn't scary enough, the executive officer told me I had no lifeboat assignment for an "abandon ship" order because the doctor was bound to stay in the medical suite until the orchestra had departed and was expected to be the second-to-last one off the ship, just before the captain.

One Sunday, on our first stop at a foreign port, I decided to go ashore in one of the vessel's tenders for sightseeing, while the nurse remained aboard to handle any medical problems arising among the few passengers who hadn't disembarked. That town was notable for a club named Senor Juan's Cantina, which I visited to buy a souvenir T-shirt for a young friend, a neighbor. He had asked me to get one with the Senor Juan's logo so he could impress his friends at his favorite watering holes back home by claiming he had "been there, done that, and got the T-shirt."

It was midmorning when I reached Senor Juan's. I found the place in a disheveled, chaotic state, from the events of the Saturday night before. Everything was in disarray—chairs knocked over, a table overturned. The floor was wet from many spilled drinks and littered with broken glass, paper napkins, and cigarette butts. The whole place reeked of booze, sweat, and cigarette smoke.

The bar and back bar had just been cleaned and restocked by the sole employee on the premises. He sold me the T-shirt with the Senor Juan's logo.

I then continued my sightseeing tour of this quaint, scenic, little village, before returning to the ship to don my white officer's uniform with red epaulets. My wife and I would be joining the captain as guests at his table for dinner.

Our ship was scheduled to depart for the next port at sunset. However, at sailing time, a number of the younger passengers who had gone ashore had not yet returned. The captain, becoming more and more distressed as the time to sail approached and then passed, periodically blew the ship's whistle, which was loud enough to be heard all across the little town. Just as the captain announced, "The crew will stand by to cast off," several taxis rolled up. About twenty singing, laughing, shouting, swearing youths spilled out of the cabs and onto the dock and then staggered toward our gangway, waving and shouting at their friends and relatives already aboard. These and all of the other passengers were lined up along the rails to watch as the big ship left the dock and sailed off into the sunset, and were now treated to the amusing spectacle below.

But for the doctor and nurse, it was just the beginning of a nightmarish evening.

Over the next few hours, the ship's nurse and I were repeatedly paged by the friends and families of these young revelers, with urgent requests for cabin calls. As I went from cabin to cabin, I heard a similar story. The young partiers' behavior was extremely bizarre after returning to their staterooms. There seemed to be no way to calm their agitation or "high," or to restrain them. I was often asked to administer some kind of tranquilizer or sleeping medication to quiet the young person down until he or she could behave normally. One young man's father told me that his son was tremulous, acting out outrageously, and hallucinating after spending the afternoon and early evening at Senor Juan's Cantina. Upon his return to the ship, the young man did not seem to know or recognize his parents and was also confused as to the time of day and his whereabouts. He was so demented that he pulled open his underwear drawer, mistook it for a toilet, and defecated into the drawer. He then ran out of the cabin and disappeared down the hallway.

In spite of the best efforts of their family members and friends, these boisterous merrymakers kept the ship's security personnel busy the rest of the night. Luckily, there were no serious injuries or fatalities, and no one fell overboard. Next day, all were accounted for, but most remained in their staterooms all day, probably with their worst-ever hangovers.

During my tour of duty, the ship docked at the seaport where Senor Juan's Cantina was situated twice more, each visit being a repeat of the first!

When the ship's regular doctor returned to duty, I asked him about the bizarre behavior of the young passengers and the incidents that went beyond drunkenness. He informed me that he suspected that this bar routinely spiked the patrons' drinks with something. He believed it was absinthe, known in nineteenth-century France as the highly alcoholic drink that makes one crazy. If that were so, an alcoholic drink mixed with absinthe would alter a person's behavior, and perceptions, much as LSD would. Sadly, it has made this now-infamous bar a lucrative tourist attraction for cruise ship passengers.

Absinthe is a clear green liqueur that was in vogue during La Belle Époque, an era of peace and plenty from 1890 to 1914 in Paris. Its popularity as a mind-altering beverage spread to other cities in Europe and America.

The principal ingredient of absinthe is a volatile oil derived from the leaves and flower heads of the perennial herb wormwood *(Artemisia absinthium)*. Other common ingredients are anise, fennel, juniper, and a variety of herbs.

Part of the appeal of absinthe during La Belle Époque was the ritual performed before imbibing it. Absinthe was served in a special glass along with a decanter of cold water and a perforated spoon containing a lump of sugar. As one poured the water over the sugar into the glass, the clear green liqueur changed to a beautiful opalescent yellow. When the drink was sipped in small quantities, it provided a pleasurable high. It was the favorite diversion of such artists as Toulouse-Lautrec, Van Gogh, and Gauguin, all of whom depicted absinthe drinkers in their paintings. However, if the drink was consumed in excess, the drinker could experience slurred speech, agitation, trembling, hallucinations, vertigo, vomiting, diarrhea, convulsions, pulmonary edema, unconsciousness, and even death. In the early twentieth century, because of its toxicity, the production and sale of absinthe were banned in the United States and most of Europe, only becoming available again in Europe in the 1990s and in the United States in 2007. And now, perhaps Senor Juan had resurrected that libation.

Or was it just bad alcoholic behavior the youths exhibited?

CHAPTER 20

The Man Who Bent Backward In Pain

> *"See one, do one, teach one. Then you are an expert!"*
>
> —Old medical adage

PAUL WAS A likable, big, and fit thirty-year-old schoolteacher who had always enjoyed good health. He had never suffered from any significant illnesses or any known allergies to medications. When he came to our office, Paul was dehydrated and appeared seriously ill, apparently from complications of food poisoning. This illness was manifested by malaise, pyrexia (fever), myalgia (achy muscles), and cephalgia (headache), as well as repeated copious emesis (vomiting) and severe diarrhea of several days' duration.

In any acute gastrointestinal infection such as Paul's, the principal medical concern is dehydration and electrolyte imbalance (loss of equilibrium between chemicals in the blood and tissues). Since the natural secretions in the GI tract are rich in sodium chloride, potassium, and other vital substances, their loss in vomitus and liquid feces can rapidly lead to profound changes in the functioning of the various organ systems. After reviewing the history of this present illness, and performing a brief physical examination, my provisional diagnosis was acute gastroenteritis secondary to food poisoning, with complications. I recommended immediate hospitalization.

Upon admission to a hospital, Paul was started on IV fluids of hypertonic (concentrated) saline and glucose solution with the addition of potassium, to replace the chemicals he had lost. To prevent any additional loss of bodily fluids containing these necessary elements, I ordered intramuscular injections of Compazine, an antiemetic (antivomiting) medication. It is the most effective medication for the nausea and vomiting of gastrointestinal disorders that occur with food poisoning, as well as for vomiting post-op and post-chemotherapy, and with motion sickness. I also had Paul take Lomotil tablets to slow up the passage of the intestinal contents through the bowel, and thereby retard or stop his diarrhea. In the hope of eliminating the causative micro-organism of the food poisoning that started all the trouble, I prescribed an IM and oral antibiotic.

Upon checking Paul on my way home after office hours, he was much improved, and the diarrhea and vomiting had ceased.

On the second day of Paul's hospitalization, I was making rounds. During rounds, [daily visits by a physician to his or her hospitalized patients], the physician reevaluates the status of each patient and writes orders for nursing care, diet, and medication, as well as laboratory and imaging studies. As I approached the nurse's station in the wing of the hospital where Paul was quartered, an RN approached in a hurried and panicked manner. Her countenance and voice both relayed concern and stress.

She exclaimed, "Oh, Doctor, please come quickly. Your patient in room 202 is thrashing around on his bed and yelling from the pain that he is experiencing. He appears to be having severe muscle spasms, which are causing him to bend backward in his bed! Also, his eyes are rotating wildly in all directions. I've never seen anything like it!"

As we neared Paul's room, I could hear him crying out in pain. It was just as the nurse had described. Paul was lying supine on the bed with his feet and his head pressing down on the mattress, his torso and buttocks arched upward. Then he rolled onto his side with his back still severely curved forward, a posture called opisthotonos (from the Greek words *opistho* meaning trunk and *tonus* meaning muscle tension). He appeared to be having severe painful spasms of the paraspinal or extensor muscles on either side of the spine which were hyperextending the torso. This condition is often seen in cases of meningitis; however, that diagnosis did not apply in Paul's case. His condition also resembled the repetitive muscle contractions seen in grand mal seizures (convulsions), but since Paul was alert, thinking, and speaking lucidly, I quickly excluded seizures as a cause. Paul's face was contorted in a painful grimace, and his eyeballs were circling randomly in what is known as an oculogyric crisis. After admitting to the nurse that I, too, had never seen anything like this before, I immediately picked up the phone and rang the doctor's lounge. An older internist (a specialist in internal medical conditions) happened to answer. "Marty, will you please come to room 202 stat?" I asked. "I need your help!"

When Marty arrived at Paul's bedside, he needed only one glance at Paul's contortions and eyes to make a diagnosis. "He's having an idiosyncrasy reaction to Compazine," Marty said calmly. "Just give him 50 mg of Benadryl IV, and he will be all right in a few minutes. Of course, after what he's been experiencing, he will be sore all over tomorrow." Marty continued, "Such violent reactions to Compazine are exceedingly rare, so don't feel bad that you did not know what caused it. I didn't know what the hell it was either, the first time I saw it."

The RN quickly brought a syringe and needle filled with the medication ordered. She dutifully showed me the vial of Benadryl from which she had drawn the fluid so that I could read the label and held up the syringe so that I could see the dose she was preparing to administer. We applied a tourniquet to the patient's arm, causing the veins to bulge. Then I inserted the needle into a vein in Paul's forearm, released the tourniquet, and injected the medication very slowly into the vein. In a short time, as my colleague had predicted, the muscle spasms subsided, and Paul calmed down.

Several years after this incident with Paul, when I was the physician on call for our medical group one day, I received a telephone call from the ER physician at a hospital in a nearby community. He stated that a young patient of one of the physicians in our call group had just arrived by ambulance at his facility. He was calling to ask the patient's medical history to help him assess her present medical crisis. The ER doctor sounded perplexed as he told me, "I've got a thirty-five-year-old woman here who is racked with some weird seizurelike contortion that is causing her to hyperextend her entire body backward. She is lying on her side, crying out in pain due to muscle spasms so severe that her occipital region [the back of the head] is practically touching her heels." He went on to say, "Simultaneously, her extraocular muscles are causing her eye globes to gyrate. I have never seen anything like it!"

I told the doctor, "I'm not familiar with that patient's medical history, but just from your description, I can tell you her diagnosis, and how to treat it."

"I'd be grateful if you would," he replied.

"She's having an idiosyncrasy reaction to Compazine," I said calmly. "Just give her 50 mg of Benadryl IV, and she'll be all right in a few minutes. Of course, after what she has been experiencing, she will be sore all over tomorrow." I went on, "Such violent reactions to Compazine are exceedingly rare. So don't feel bad that you did not know what caused her reaction. I didn't know what the hell it was either the first time I saw it."

After a few hastily-made phone calls, I verified that my diagnosis was correct. The woman had been given Compazine for nausea that she was experiencing following an outpatient surgical procedure she had undergone that morning. When I called the ER physician back with this additional information, he said that the young woman had already responded remarkably well to the treatment I had recommended. He thanked me for my insightful diagnosis. I responded "This has been a great example of the old adage we learned at medical school. See one, do one, teach one—then you are an expert!"

This type of learning experience is something that cannot be taught at medical school because the condition is so rare that it would probably not occur during a medical student's training. The only option for a professor of medicine in teaching students about such a condition is to describe the symptoms and how to handle it. He or she can only hope that when the students are later confronted with this or similar rare syndromes, they will retrieve the lesson from their memory banks and make a correct diagnosis. Being realistic, I believe that until a physician observes at least once the clinical picture of an exceedingly rare condition, he or she will not have sufficient information to recognize it.

CHAPTER 21

The Man Who Couldn't Pee

TIM, AN EASYGOING man in late middle age, was returning from a coast-to-coast business trip. He had been unable to urinate first thing upon arising at his hotel that morning which seemed strange. He assumed that at some point while showering, dressing, and packing he would have no trouble emptying his bladder. But he was unable to do so. Nor was he able to go at the New York airport before takeoff. During the flight home, he visited the restroom a few times, but he couldn't get a stream started, either standing up or sitting down. His lower abdomen began to hurt, and he began to worry. As the hours passed, his overfull bladder became so painful that he wondered if it was going to burst! He wisely drank no fluids, but couldn't help fidgeting and squirming for the rest of the long flight.

He was able to call his wife from his mobile phone and ask her to pick him up at the airport and take him straight to his doctor's office.

He even asked the hostess to let him go through first class after landing so that he could be the first passenger off the aircraft. Tim took time to try again at a men's room on his way to the baggage carousel, but he still could not pee.

Meanwhile, his wife had called our office to ask if she could bring him there for relief of this problem, although they would not arrive until shortly after our usual closing time. The office staff reassured her that the doctor would wait. I spoke with her and asked her if she was aware of him taking antihistamine tablets for allergy. She said, "Yes, he bought some yesterday for a flare-up in his hay fever."

"That's what triggered his urine retention problem," I replied. "But there is an underlying cause we'll need to look into later."

Upon their arrival at my office, I injected lidocaine gel as an anesthetic and a lubricant down the opening at the tip of his penis, then slid a plastic catheter into and down through the urethra, the bladder outlet tube that runs through the penis. It had to be painfully forced past the obstruction, which was due to enlargement of the prostate gland that surrounds the urethra at the bladder outlet. This allowed the bladder to be slowly drained through the catheter of a near-record amount of urine, much to the relief of the tortured patient, who blurted out, "Oh, that felt so good, as soon as the urine started running!"

The catheter was left in place, and the nurse connected it to a long plastic tube leading to a urine-collecting bag she taped to his leg, which went everywhere he went for the next day or two.

I explained to the patient and his wife that all men in midlife begin to get a slowly progressive enlargement of their prostate gland which, because of its anatomical location surrounding the urethra, eventually constricts the bladder outlet.

When I reviewed with Tim his urinary history, he described the classic group of gradually occurring symptoms of prostate enlargement: increasing frequency of bathroom visits, taking longer to initiate urination, smaller caliber of urine stream, bladder taking longer to empty, and having to strain hard to force the last little bit out, then passing gas simultaneously.

This constellation of symptoms inexorably occurs in every man as he ages. It also can lead to residual urine after voiding, leaving the same old bacteria to multiply, which is the primary cause of acute and chronic cystitis (bladder infection) and nephritis (kidney infection).

In Tim's case, the inability to void was mostly due to his underlying prostate gland enlargement slowly constricting his urethra. But it was triggered by a side effect of taking an antihistamine capsule for his respiratory allergy: diminished force of bladder wall contractions, allowing the bladder to overfill (to over two quarts in this patient's case), which by ballooning and thinning of the bladder wall also weakened the wall muscles.

After a return visit to remove the catheter and the urine-collecting bag, I referred Tim to a urologist for follow-up. That specialist initially prescribed one of several medications capable of shrinking the prostate gland over time, allowing free flow of urine. However, in Tim's case, this treatment failed. A year later, ongoing obstruction caused a bladder and prostate infection, leading to a severe whole-body illness called sepsis (blood poisoning). A course of daily self-administered IV high-dose antibiotics was prescribed for this life-threatening infection.

That complication later required a laser "reboring" procedure, called a transurethral prostatectomy, where, under a general anesthetic, a new, larger channel was carved by way of the penile urethra, through the encircling prostate gland, into the bladder. That operation restored his normal, powerful urine flow.

Following that procedure, with follow-up antibiotic therapy, his bladder symptoms and infections never returned.

If we don't count the naughty and not-nice social diseases, the leading cause of male urinary tract infections is backing up of urine. It can happen, as we have seen, due to the prostate gland's natural enlargement with age. In other cases, such infections may occur when a kidney stone forms in the kidney, tries to pass through the urine, and then clogs the ureter. There may also be a neurologic origin, secondary to spinal-cord diseases or injuries, causing weak bladder contractions and resulting in incomplete emptying of the bladder and residual urine, where bacteria thrive and multiply exponentially.

This case history reveals what most men will experience if they live long enough: prostate gland enlargement causing urinary backing up, followed by infection of the bladder, prostate, or kidney. Such infections occasionally culminate in bacteremia (microorganisms in the blood) and sepsis, a whole-body, potentially fatal, systemic infection.

Even little precautions, such as not being too quick to zip up, can help bladder emptying. Standing at the urinal or sitting on the toilet a little longer helps expel the last few drops of urine. Also, while having a bowel movement and urinating simultaneously, men should try for a second urination after the last of the rectal contents have passed, relieving pressure on the bladder. Of course, it is essential to stay well hydrated, too. Up to two quarts of water a day is desirable to dilute urine and reduce the bacterial concentration in the urogenital system.

CHAPTER 22

The Man Who Nearly Bled To Death, And The Girl Who Did

The Man Who Nearly Bled to Death . . .

T HIS STORY CONCERNS David, a twenty-five-year-old, college-educated stockbroker who took a couple of Tylenol tablets for a gnawing pain in his epigastric (upper abdominal) region. A few hours later, the pain was still there, so he took two non-steroid anti inflamatory tablets (Ibuprofen). As the pain worsened over the next week, he foolishly upped the dose to seven or eight tablets a day. When the pain began to penetrate from his abdomen through to his upper back, he mentioned it to his wife. She apparently had more common sense than he, and immediately sent him to our office without an appointment. He told the receptionist, "I don't want to be here, but my wife made me promise to come."

After one glance at him, the nurse sat him down, then immediately went to the exam room where she knew I was attending another patient. She knocked, opened the door, said, "Excuse me," to the patient and then said to me, "Oh, Doctor, a man just walked into our waiting room looking as pale as that stiff I saw on a slab in the morgue in my training!"

I rushed out, took one look, and brought David into an empty room and helped him up onto the exam table. The nurse instantly drew blood from his arm and sent the samples through the pneumatic tube system to the hospital laboratory, requesting a stat blood count, as well as typing and cross matching for a blood transfusion.

As I gently palpated his upper abdomen and epigastrium, just over his stomach and just below the sternum, it was exquisitely tender to light touch. But there were no other significant findings, except for his apparent generalized weakness.

I asked if his bowel movements had been a black color. He said, "Like tar, for a week."

I asked if he had taken a lot of aspirin. He said, "No, but I had to take a lot of Advil for the pain."

I told him, "My god! You have burned a hole in the delicate lining of the back of your your stomach, causing a penetrating bleeding ulcer. You are lucky that the ulcer eroded only a small blood vessel rather than a large one, enabling you to adapt as the quantity of circulating blood became smaller and smaller. Now, you have gradually lost almost all of your blood. But don't worry, we can get an expert doctor to slide a gastroscope down your throat into the stomach, where the ulcer can be seen and cauterized. Simultaneously you will receive transfusions of blood that has already been matched to yours, and you will be back to normal in no time!"

Our receptionist, meanwhile, on her own initiative had phoned a couple of my favorite gastroenterologists, to ask their locations. One of them happened to be in the adjacent hospital. When apprised of our emergency, he said, "Wheel him right down to the ER. I will meet him there where we will fill up his near-empty bloodstream with the blood you ordered, scope him, and stop the bleed right away!"

So we put him in a wheelchair, and my receptionist wheeled him to the elevator and down to the ER only a few yards away.

Minutes later the lab returned the patient's CBC showing his hemoglobin (oxygen-carrying component of red blood cells), to be only 4.5 grams per deciliter, on a scale where normal is 12 to 14 grams and anything less than 5 grams is inconsistent with life. But since the patient had walked into our office on his own, it meant that his young, healthy, amazing body had adapted to some extent to his ongoing blood loss.

The gastroenterologist called later to say all had gone well with his procedure, the gastric mucous membrane was terribly inflamed. He found the ulcer on the back of his stomach and was able to cauterize it, and staunch the hemorrhage. He then said that my staff and I had saved another one.

After seeing a few more patients, I went down to the ER to visit the patient, who now had received four units of blood, and was pink again. When he thanked me, I said, "No, thank your wife. It was her female intuition that saved your life!"

He came back to our office two days later, to thank my staff, who were surprised that he could look so healthy again so fast.

He told us he had done research and was astounded to learn that eighteen thousand Americans die each year from a bleeding ulcer, mostly caused by aspirin and NSAIDs like Ibuprofen when labeled dosages are exceeded.

I would add this warning for my readers: anyone who takes aspirin, even at the recommended dose, for three weeks *will* get a stomach ulcer, though not necessarily a bleeding ulcer.

. . . *And the Girl Who Did*

This is a sad but true story about the sudden death of a teenage girl who did not have to die but did—because of the ignorance of bystanders who called 911 but did not know the basic principles of first aid.

She was not my patient, and I was not present, but I read about it in the local newspaper. I know a reliable source who had been there. This is her recollection: "It was at a pool party for a Girl Scout troop on a beautiful hot summer day. The unfortunate girl went from the pool apron into the house without realizing that the sliding glass door into the dining room was closed, and she walked right through it." Apparently, the glass was not tempered, so instead of shattering into a thousand little pieces, it came crashing down as a guillotine-like sheet of glass, severing an artery in her upper thigh. A large artery in the pelvis, the iliac artery, extends from the body's main artery, the aorta, and becomes the femoral artery that supplies blood to the leg. One of one of those large arteries must have been sliced. With every beat of her heart, the girl's lifeblood pumped out onto the dining room floor. Tragically, not a single person who was there that day knew that by just applying direct pressure to the wound until help arrived, they could have saved her life. Any gentleman present could have taken his folded handkerchief and pressed it on the bleeding site with the heel of his hand until the paramedics came and put a clamp on the bleeder.

CHAPTER 23

The Men Who Can't Get It Up

T HIS IS A story of great importance to 40 percent of men aged forty; 50 percent of men aged fifty; 60 percent of men aged sixty; 70 percent of men aged seventy; and 80 percent of men aged eighty—because they all have some degree of erectile dysfunction.

Once in a while, *all* men have a little difficulty obtaining or maintaining an erection and achieving an orgasm. However, if a man has a consistent inability to accomplish satisfactory sexual intercourse, it is called impotence.

Because many impotent men are reluctant to talk about their problem with their spouses, significant others, girlfriends, or even with their doctors, the true prevalence of this condition is unknown. But it is estimated that ten to thirty million Americans now suffer from this ego-deflating, often embarrassing, marriage-troubling problem.

The principal reason that doctors frequently miss the diagnosis of impotence is that many patients present with other complaints, yet have this as a hidden agenda, and it doesn't surface. However, if the doctor wisely poses the question as part of a routine medical-history taking, men will often admit to the problem. Once the problem comes to light, the doctor can then take the first step to help solve the problem by assuring the patient that he is not alone with this problem, help him gain an understanding of the many possible underlying causes that must be looked for and addressed, and then reassure the patient that various treatments are available and that he doesn't have to "live with it."

In the recent past, the medical community had little understanding of this condition. It was believed that impotence was mostly due to psychological factors, such as stress, anxiety, or depression. More recently, however, scientific investigation of the subject has proven that approximately 50 to 70 percent of all cases have physical causes or a combination of both physical and psychosomatic causes. To appreciate how medical conditions can result in impotence, a brief review of the complex anatomy (structure) and physiology (functioning) of the male genital system is in order.

The testicles and adrenals (small glands adjacent to the kidneys that secrete many different hormones) both secrete the male hormone testosterone into the bloodstream daily. The presence of this hormone is the basis of all things male, including libido, so that visual, auditory, and tactile cues, as well as thoughts and fantasies, bring about arousal. This causes the brain to transmit electrical impulses down the spinal cord to the pelvic outflow of the spinal nerves into the genital region. These signals bring about muscle relaxation within the walls of the arteries supplying blood to the penis, allowing those vessels to dilate and pump blood under pressure into the corpora cavernosa. The organ then becomes rigid, as the veins which normally drain blood out of the penis are closed off by the increasing hydraulic arterial pressure.

In such a complex system, a malfunction at any level can cause ED, rendering the man impotent.

The most common cause of impotence is atherosclerosis, a lifelong build-up of calcified fat deposits in the lining of all arteries in the body, related to inheritance, but caused primarily by hypertension, hyperlipidemia, smoking, and diabetes. The same arteriosclerotic process that eventually narrows and clogs the coronary arteries, leading to heart attack, or clogs the carotid arteries in the neck or the cerebral arteries, leading to a stroke, can narrow or clog the arteries supplying blood to the penis. This means that any man experiencing ED should have a complete workup by a doctor looking for early signs of heart disease as well as looking into other causes of impotence.

Psychological causes that may inhibit arousal include anxiety or depressive reaction caused by emotional stress, negative thoughts such as guilt, or "it didn't work last time, I wonder if it'll work this time." Any neurological disorder, such as multiple sclerosis, amyotrophic lateral sclerosis (Lou Gehrig's disease), diabetic neuropathy, or a spinal-cord injury or tumor, can interfere with nerve conduction down the spinal cord. Yet another common cause of impotence is side effects of prescription medications, and a few over-the-counter medications acting centrally in the brain can inhibit initiation of the cascade of neurological events or affect the vascular system, impairing blood flow to the genitals.

Men with impotence must swallow their macho pride and talk to their physicians if they have this problem. The physician, of course, will listen carefully to the patient's complaints, take a careful medical and surgical history, and inquire about medications being taken. The physician will then perform a physical examination with special attention to the nervous system, the cardiovascular system, the genitals, and the prostate gland.

If it becomes apparent that medication is causing the impotence, alternate medications can be found. If there appears to be a psychosomatic cause, the patient will be treated with medical therapy, such as tranquilizers or antidepressants, or he may be referred to a psychiatrist or clinical psychologist.

On the other hand, if a physiological or anatomical cause is established, the patient will likely be referred to a urologist. Following the urologist's own history taking and physical examination to rule out cancer or other serious conditions, he or she may evaluate the patient by means of a special device that fits over the patient's penis during sleep to monitor nocturnal erections. Only after this thorough investigation will treatment be recommended.

LAWRENCE R. BROWNLEE, M.D.

There are a variety of treatments for erectile dysfunction:

1. Mechanical
    a. Elastic ring around the base of the penis, to prevent outflow of blood
    b. Vacuum device, to draw blood into the penis
2. Pharmacologic
    a. Oral tablets (e.g., Cialis)
    b. Testosterone (topical gel or skin patch applied daily)
    c. Intramuscular depo-testosterone injection every three weeks
    d. Self-injection of medication into the penile shaft, just prior to intercourse
3. Surgical [see also, Chapter 12]
    a. Penile shaft implant
    b. Hydraulic scrotum and shaft implants
    c. Vascular surgery

When the response to the first few, conservative measures is disappointing, a few patients will try self-injection of a pharmacologic agent, such as papaverine, directly into the penile shaft each time, prior to anticipated intercourse. This causes increased blood flow into the dorsal arteries of the penis, resulting in a good, lasting erection. The disadvantages of this method are apprehension and mild local pain at the site of the injection, as well as possible priapism (prolonged painful erection even after orgasm). This

192

method also has the potential for permanent fibrosis (scarring).

If the patient chooses the noninvasive option of a vacuum erection device, there are several brands available on the market. The flaccid penis is inserted into the open end of a clear plastic cylinder, and a hand-operated pump evacuates the air, allowing the penis to fill with blood until it is engorged, at which time a special elastic band is slipped off the cylinder and around the base of the penis, preventing outflow of the blood and maintaining the erection until afterward, when the rubber band is removed.

When all of these relatively inexpensive and relatively safe options have been tried and found unhelpful or undesirable, the patient may choose the ultimate solution—a surgically implanted prosthesis or the more complex hydraulic prosthesis. While the latter procedure is the most expensive, most complex, and most invasive, it is perhaps the most effective solution to the ED problem. Tens of thousands of this type of hydraulic penile prosthesis have been implanted. They achieve near-natural erectile function, are aesthetically pleasing, complications are rare, and mechanical failure in the newer versions is exceedingly rare and can often be corrected with only minor outpatient surgery.

If the man was able to achieve orgasm and ejaculation prior to the surgical procedure but lacked an erection, he will be able to climax post-op as well. Most couples choosing this option find this to be an ideal solution to impotence.

CHAPTER 24

The Airline Pilot Who Took Too Many Health Food Supplements

W HEN PETER, AN experienced thirty-seven-year-old commercial airline pilot, signed in as a new patient at our front desk, the receptionist asked what condition he wished to see the doctor about.

He replied, "I have a health problem which is affecting my work. I have seen my regular physician, who tried his best but was stumped. He referred me to a specialist, who was unable to solve my problem either. I have now been referred here by my neighbor, a heart-and-lung surgeon who said your doctor is a good diagnostician."

After Peter completed his paperwork, including his past medical/surgical history and current prescription medications and names of nutrition supplements, the nurse knew this would require a comprehensive physical examination, so she performed the preliminary tasks of height, weight, blood pressure, heart rate, body mass index, and Mini-Mental Status Exam. She then took Peter to an examining room, gave him a paper gown, suggested he strip to his underwear, and said, "The doctor will be with you shortly. Meanwhile would you please do these self tests for anxiety and depression."

She then came to me and said, "Wow! This is going to be a real challenge, Doctor."

After introducing myself to Peter, I sat down to chitchat briefly about his work, life, and family, and answered his questions about my medical training, experience, etc. I then turned to review the past medical, surgical, and family history, list of prescription (Rx) medicine, and information on hobbies he had written down. He proudly said he was healthy and fit from being an avid mountain biker and required no prescription medication but took a few health foods.

I asked him to describe the vexing problem that had caused him to ask his employer for three weeks of sick leave from his commercial-airline pilot duties.

He said, "Following five years as a copilot, and ten years' experience as a captain flying everything from prop jets to twin-engine and four-engine jets, I believed I was the best pilot in the fleet. I was calm and self-confident to the point of cockiness. I could make landings so smooth, passengers frequently commented on it as they deplaned. But a couple of months ago, I became very nervous, finding myself double-checking all controls, gauges, and switches. I was so tremulous it felt like I had a motor going inside me that I couldn't shut off." He went on to say,

"I was actually trembling as I pulled the yoke back, causing vibration on takeoff, and I was making hard landings too. When several copilots mentioned it, I knew that for safety, I must book off for several weeks until I sorted it out."

I proceeded to make a meticulous, prolonged physical examination but found no significant abnormalities in any organ system. This was followed by a comprehensive battery of laboratory studies; all of which proved to be normal.

At the follow-up visit in a few days later, while showing him the results of all of our tests, I asked further questions. One of which was, "You said you took a few health foods and you listed five. Can you give me the names of some of any others?"

Peter produced a list of twenty-four over-the-counter "health" supplements that he took daily! He said, "I have to shop at several different nutrition stores to find them all."

I said, "Pete, we have found our diagnosis. I can't tell you which, but at least one item on that list must be responsible for the way you feel. It's probably something that has caffeinelike or thyroidlike properties, and that is making you nervous and shaky. So all you have to do is stop the health foods, and you will return to normal very quickly."

He responded, "But, Doctor, I shouldn't have to stop them all. Why can't we eliminate just a few that are the most likely to cause my symptoms?"

"No, Pete. You've heard the old adage, 'one man's meat is another man's poison.' You must stop them all. Please ask my receptionist to give you an appointment for seven to ten days from now, and at that time, I will be able to give you a release to let you return to work," I said calmly and confidently, "almost to the point of cockiness" (to use his expression).

Later that day, I showed a specialist I shared the office with the list of health foods the patient had been on.

"That's nothing," he said. "I have a lady patient who was taking forty nutritional pills a day and was wondering why she didn't feel well!"

Peter returned ten days later. With a big smile, he said, "You were right, Doc, it only took three or four days to feel normal again after quitting all that health-food stuff, so I went back to flying and mountain biking. I didn't need a doctor's note because the first day back to the airline, I volunteered to have our check pilot check me out in the flight simulator, and I passed easily. But today I had the best test of all. Returning to our local airport in a heavy Boeing 737 aircraft, we encountered a wind-shear situation, where on approach for a landing the wind suddenly changed direction from a forty-knot headwind to a tailwind, and suddenly, we didn't have enough airspeed to stay aloft. So I immediately and calmly applied full thrust and rotated the aircraft up to stick shaker, a stall-warning attitude, to regain the loss of altitude until the airspeed recovered. We then conducted a missed-approach procedure, raising the landing gear and adjusting the flap setting to twenty degrees.

Consequently, we did a circling approach to an into-the-wind, stabilized landing carried out safely."

Then Peter, the airline captain who had wisely suspended himself from flying when he knew he wasn't himself, gratefully presented me with a gift certificate for my wife and me to have dinner at the finest restaurant in the city. I thanked him and thought to myself: "Twenty four supplements, and the experts couldn't solve this problem. Duh!"

CHAPTER 25

Patients With Foreign Objects In Them

The Boy Who Drove a Toy Car into His Nose

Accoording to the history of the present illness (HPI) the nurse had recorded on the boy's chart, his mother had reported he'd had clear mucus running from his nose for a week.

"Then the snot turned thick and green," and two days later, he became sick and feverish.

The nurse had noted a temp of 102°F.

After reading the HPI and entering the exam room, I greeted the mother, then turned to the little five-year-old patient sitting on the end of the examining table. With one glance, I could see he was very ill. He looked droopy, his skin was pale, his face was flushed, and his eyes looked tired. The left side of the boy's nose and left cheek were swollen and red.

I smiled and said to him, "What is your name, sonny?"

He told me his name was William. I asked if that was what I should call him, and he said, "Well, everybody calls me Billy."

"Okay, Billy," I said, "I need to look in your nose with this bright light I am putting on my forehead. But first, I will swab your nose gently with a Q-tip and a little magic jelly that will stop it from hurting. Then I will spread your nose open a little wider with this instrument to get a good look inside."

"Okay," he said bravely.

A few minutes later, I spotted the obstruction. Inserting forceps and probing the object, I found it to be metal. I was able to grasp it and slowly pull it out, followed by a copious flow of purulent (pussy) discharge. His mom gasped, and the nurse said "Wow" when I displayed a miniature toy car!

"What a good boy you are, Billy, for making it easy for me to help you," I said.

The nurse lavaged the nostrils clear with warm, sterile water, gauze, and cotton swabs while I examined Billy's other organ systems and wrote a prescription for cherry-flavored antibiotic syrup.

The surprised and much-relieved mother was asked to make an appointment at the front desk for a follow-up in three days, but she was cautioned to call earlier if Billy became any sicker. When I saw Billy three days later, all the swelling had subsided and he looked healthy and energetic and ready for his next adventure.

The Fisherman Who Hooked Himself

Harold, an avid fly fisherman, stood happily in his hip waders with water up to his knees on the shore of a fast-moving mountain stream. He was hoping to catch a steelhead trout. Harold became excited when on his first cast it felt as if a fish had taken the hook. For a moment, he felt and saw nothing; then suddenly he saw a splash and felt the familiar tug on his line of a fish trying to run with the hook, and he knew he had caught a big one—perhaps too big for the light nylon line he was using. He knew he would have to keep the tip of his rod up and reel the line in a little whenever his quarry gave him a little slack. Man and beast battled, until the line suddenly snapped, at which time Jack felt a slap on the side of his face. He knew then that instead of having fish for dinner, this would become one of those tall-tales about the one that got away.

Several weeks later, Jack was in my office relating his story. Recently he had noted what he thought was a pimple on his cheek, which soon enlarged, the skin around it growing swollen and red.

"Yesterday it developed this bubble with yellow liquid under it," he told me.

"Well, you were wise to come in for treatment," I said, "because an infection such as this must be opened and drained, or it will not heal. So I'll ask the nurse to prepare a minor-surgery tray so we can do an incision-and-drainage procedure."

After making a small incision in the dome over the lesion, as expected malodorous pus squirted out. It was blotted with gauze, then I could see something green In the crater. Using forceps I grasped it and slowly pulled out a coiled up four-inch long nylon fishing line!

The nurse said wow! The patient said what is it? I said it's the most unusual foreign body I have ever found in a patient. And it explains the slap in the face that you felt when you're fishing line broke under high tension. I completed the procedure, dressed the wound, and sent Harold along with my wishes for a better catch on his next fishing adventure.

The Lady Who Forgot a Tampon

Our hallway signal system showed that the next patient was ready for me. As customary, I took the patient's chart from the door pocket and glanced at the nurse's notes. The patient was the forty-one-year-old woman who was here for her annual breast exam and mammogram as well as pelvic organ exam and Pap smear. Her last menstrual period had been three weeks before. As usual, the patient was reclining on the table in a pink paper gown with a paper sheet over her legs which were up in stirrups. After greeting her and taking my seat on the stool at the bottom of the table, she said, "Oh! By the way, doctor, a coworker and several friends have mentioned that I have unpleasant body odor. I was already showering every day, so then I began tub baths, but it didn't help. It's not underarm BO. My friends said to ask my doctor."

"Thanks for that information. I will keep that in mind as I examine you," I told her. After inspecting the external genitalia and anus, I inserted an illuminated speculum (a duck-bill shaped instrument) to view the interior of her vagina and to take a Pap smear from the cervical opening with a specially designed stick. I could see a foreign object in the cul-de-sac surrounding the cervix. It was an old tampon from her last menses several weeks ago. I used forceps to grasp it and remove it along with a thick covering of malodorous, discolored secretions, then sealed it in a sterile plastic bag to be sent to a lab for bacterial analysis. The remaining fluids were wiped with large cotton swabs then sealed in a plastic bag and put in the trash for special handling. Of course, she needed a vaginal douche afterward with an antiseptic solution. The douching was carried out by the nurse and our back-office assistant, also a female employee, to minimize the patient's embarrassment. We then opened the windows, mopped the floor, sterilized the instruments, and sealed the room off temporarily until it had fully aired out.

Upon recheck a few days later, the patient's vaginal tissues and cervix appeared normal and her vaginal secretions were clear and odorless. We told her how fortunate she was not to have incurred a life-threatening pelvic-organ infection from her forgotten tampon, because, as it turned out, the lab had reported that her specimen contained a flesh-eating bacteria that was running rampant at that time all over North America.

She responded that she planned to continue going to church.

The Lady with a Fly in Her Ear

While on duty as the ER physician at a nearby hospital one evening, I heard a woman screaming, and then saw her dancing around and waving her arms as she jumped out of an ambulance at the rear entrance. Suddenly she halted, composed herself, and entered the room calmly. She submitted to the paperwork and then was seated on a gurney and wheeled into a cubical, where a nurse and I joined her for an examination. Just as she began to explain herself, she "freaked out" again, and had to be restrained. And again, just as suddenly she stopped. This time she had time to tell us that every few minutes she experienced an unbearable buzzing sound and vibration in her right ear and head.

I quickly grabbed an otoscope and looked into her right ear. I was astounded to see a housefly silhouetted against the patient's tympanic membrane. I guess my examination disturbed the fly, because it started flapping its wings against her eardrum, and she went nuts again.

I called for an ear syringe, a water source, and a kidney-shaped basin to do an ear lavage. As I squirted the warm water into her external auditory canal, it would hit the tympanic membrane and flow back out. On the second or third squirt, the offending housefly appeared in the basin!

I have never had a more thankful patient.

The Marine Who Coughed Up Rusty Shrapnel

A longtime patient of mine, Barnaby was a retired Marine who had seen action in the Pacific Theater in World War II. On this occasion, he presented at my office with a chesty cough productive of copious amounts of purulent sputum (mucus). He also complained of chest pain, malaise, and a fever, all of which had been present for three or four days.

The nurse found his blood pressure was good at 120/70, but his temperature was 103°F.

I systematically examined his skin, eyes, ears, nose, and throat and found only moderate redness in his pharynx and nares.

Pulling my stethoscope out of my jacket pocket (only TV docs and wannabe docs hang stethoscopes around their necks), I listened to his lungs. I heard the typical coarse, musical sounds of rhonchi, indicating the presence of thick mucus scattered throughout his bronchial tubes in both lung fields. But more importantly, I heard rales—the soft, subtle sounds of pneumonia—in his left lower lung field.

Chest radiographs were taken on the premises. Looking at the films on my view box a few minutes later, I could detect a significant white patch in the lower lobe of the left lung. It had a central core a half inch in diameter, possibly a cancerous tumor. But it was so dense it could even be metal. Whatever it was, it was blocking a sizeable bronchial tube, which was the etiology of his pneumonia.

For treatment of Barnaby's lung infection, there was a choice of several antibiotics. In the early 1900s pneumonia was the number-one cause of death in the world, because antibiotics like sulfa and penicillin were not to be invented until just before World War II. Because of the triumph of medical science over disease in the mid and late twentieth century, this patient could be easily cured.

We gave him an appointment for follow-up in several days, at which time auscultation of his chest with a stethoscope revealed partial resolution of the sounds heard earlier; he was much improved overall. I asked Barnaby to return in a month for a repeat chest X-ray, to be sure that his lungs were clear. If not, we would have to scan him for possible lung cancer.

When Barnaby returned, his lung had fully cleared up. He had brought with him a rusty piece of steel that he had coughed up. Its nature was no mystery: during the war, a Japanese hand-grenade had exploded near him. He'd had multiple minor surgeries to remove all the shrapnel, but the doctors had missed this piece!

The Man with a Glass Stirring Rod in His Penis

Fanny and Fred were famous partiers, drinkers, and hell-raisers in their social circle.

Following an evening of dining, dancing, imbibing, and making whoopee, they managed to find their way home and had relations. An hour or so later, Fred wanted to try a second time, but could not rise to the occasion. It was Fanny's idea to try straightening him out by inserting a long glass stirring rod from her drink in Fred's urethral opening and down the length of his urethra.

At his first attempt to penetrate, the rod broke, and Fred yelled out in pain. Fanny managed to remove the last half of the glass rod, but then a lot of blood spurted out. Fanny wrapped a clean handkerchief around his penis, and he squeezed it throughout the ambulance ride to the ER.

I received Fred as the ER doctor that night and immediately called a urologist and explained the situation. The urologist said it would be best to notify the operating room that we would be opening the urethra, removing the rod and glass fragments, and doing a surgical repair within the hour. After alerting the operating room, I was able to get another doctor to come and replace me while I assisted the surgeon.

Fortunately, all went well in the procedure, but only time would tell if the resulting scar tissue in the urethra would cause urinary obstruction in the future, which often occurs when the urethra is damaged.

$\mathcal{A}$bout the Author

D R. BROWNLEE'S JOURNEY from high school drop-out to Doctor of the Year began in Regina, Saskatchewan, Canada.

Born to an American mother and Canadian father, he grew up in Saskatchewan during the depression in a poor, but close family, the youngest of six children.

As a youth, Larry found hockey, football, and dating more compelling than scholarship. Failing twelfth grade, he quit school and began working at a variety of manual labor jobs.

At age nineteen, Larry moved with his family to Victoria, British Columbia. He soon met Ilaria Bet, a student R.N., and they married six months later. Together, they self-built the house of their dreams, on a hilltop with a sea view.

But after completion of the home, he became restless and sought vocational counseling. He was advised to quit his job, go to university, and then go to medical school. A daunting, ten-year task!

So at age twenty-nine, married with a child, Larry chose scholarship over a professional football contract offer. Ilaria offered to work to put him through pre-med studies at UCLA, followed by medical school at the University of British Columbia in Vancouver, B.C., Canada..

After he had earned his M.D. degree, and lured by the southern California climate, Larry, his wife, and their three daughters emigrated to Orange County, California, where he pursued post-graduate training at the University of California, Irvine.

For the next forty-three years, Dr. Brownlee enjoyed his solo Family Practice in Tustin, California, where patients, fellow physicians, nurses, and employees at their local hospital once honored him as Doctor of the Year.

Dr. Brownlee and Ilaria, his wife of sixty-four happy years of marriage, are now retired in Newport Beach, Ca.

CPSIA information can be obtained
at www.ICGtesting.com
Printed in the USA
FSHW010706231218
54655FS